YOHANN AUCANTE

THE SWEDISH EXPERIMENT

The COVID-19 Response and its Controversies

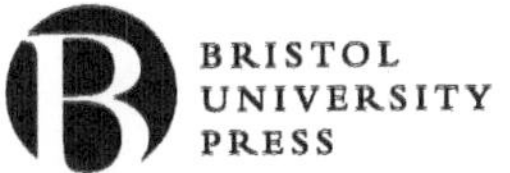
BRISTOL
UNIVERSITY
PRESS

First published in Great Britain in 2022 by

Bristol University Press
University of Bristol
1–9 Old Park Hill
Bristol
BS2 8BB
UK
t: +44 (0)117 374 6645
e: bup-info@bristol.ac.uk

Details of international sales and distribution partners are available at
bristoluniversitypress.co.uk

British Library Cataloguing in Publication Data
A catalogue record for this book is available from the British Library

ISBN 978-1-5292-2387-3 hardcover
ISBN 978-1-5292-2388-0 ePub
ISBN 978-1-5292-2389-7 ePdf

Cover design: blu inc
Front cover image: Beyhes Evren/iStock

Printed and bound by CPI Group (UK) Ltd, Croydon, CR0 4YY

Contents

List of Abbreviations

ECDC	European Centre for Disease Prevention and Control
FHM	Fokhälsomyndigheten (Swedish Public Health Agency)
GAVI	Global Alliance for Vaccines
IVO	Inspektionen för vård och omsorg (Health and Social Care Inspectorate)
LO	Landsorganisationen (Swedish Workers Trade Unions Confederation)
MSB	Myndighet för samhällskydd och Beredskap (Civil Contingency Agency)
NHS	National Health Service (UK)
OECD	Organization for Economic Cooperation and Development
SAGE	Scientific Advisory Group for Emergencies (UK)
SARS	Severe Acute Respiratory Syndrome
SD	SverigeDemokraterna (Sweden Democrats)
SS	Socialstyrelsen (National Board for Health and Welfare)
WHO	World Health Organization

About the Author

Yohann Aucante is Senior Lecturer in Politics at the School of Advanced Studies in the Social Sciences (EHESS) in Paris, France. His research focusses on Nordic politics and comparative welfare policies. He has recently published 'Paradoxes of hegemony: Scandinavian social democracy and the state', in M. Fulla, M. Lazar (eds) *European Socialists and the State* (Palgrave Macmillan, 2020) and co-directed a documentary film, *Icelandic Revolutions*, on the political consequences of the Icelandic financial crisis that was selected for the Reykjavik film festival (Aucante and Aucante, 2017). He is joint editor-in-chief of the French interdisciplinary journal of Nordic studies (*Nordiques*).

Acknowledgements

The author would like to extend his thanks to Greg Epp for helping with editing this manuscript, and Luc Foisneau, Patrick Hassenteufel, Carl Marklund and the anonymous reviewers for valuable advice. Thanks shall also go to the members of the jury d'habilitation à diriger des recherches who reviewed this work, Shirin Ahlbäck Öberg, Olivier Borraz, Nicholas Aylott, Bruno Palier and Anne Rasmussen.

Introduction

In early March 2021, when most of Western Europe and many other regions of the world were shutting down for fear of the new coronavirus, one country in the Baltic region opted for an alternative and risky pathway. Sweden, with the lowest hospital bed capacity per capita of the OECD (Organisation for Economic Cooperation and Development), went on with life – not exactly as usual, but keeping primary and middle schools open and not closing bars, restaurants, cinemas, shops or museums. Ski resorts continued to run until the end of March, and national borders remained open for a full month. Even the final round of selection for the Eurovision song contest, the highly popular Melodifestivalen, went ahead in front of a roaring crowd on 7 March, whereas the Danish counterpart had played before empty seats. During a press conference on 6 March the director of the Public Health Agency (Folkhälsomyndigheten, hereafter FHM), Johan Carlsson, said that the situation was under control in Sweden, yet two days later Italy locked down 17 million people in its northern regions, extending the measure to the entire country on 10 March. On 11 March, the World Health Organization (WHO) declared a state of pandemic of which Europe was the epicentre.

As most European countries closed their borders and implemented more or less strict lockdowns of their population (the UK being one of the last to do so), the Swedish situation started to appear as a visible anomaly, even at home. The rest of the Nordic countries adopted more stringent policies early on, although the Danish chief epidemiologist was not in favour of the strict lockdown that the government of Social Democrat Mette Frederiksen decided to implement in all haste. It is not the case that Sweden did nothing, as many foreign observers seemed to believe at the time. The authorities in charge of the crisis held daily press meetings; they advised people to wash their hands, keep their distance, stay at home in case of any symptoms and work remotely when possible; and they requested a cap of 500 people for gatherings (down to 50 by the end of March). Universities and high schools converted to distance learning. On 17 March the prime minister, Social Democrat Stefan Löfven, gave an unusual six-minute address to the nation to communicate the gravity of the situation and to urge compliance with public health recommendations. It should be added that fighting a crisis of such magnitude required more than health-related measures: the waiting period for sickness benefits was eliminated right away so that people with symptoms could stay home, and people who could not work started to receive at least partial compensation.

Within a few days, the Swedes and the rest of the world became more familiar with the very phlegmatic man who assumed the role of 'state epidemiologist', Anders Tegnell, but also to some extent with one of his predecessors in this function, his mentor Johan Giesecke, who came back from retirement to act as consultant for FHM. They both argued in favour of a piecemeal, evidence-based approach, a mitigation strategy that would imply living with the virus, as they believed that it would inevitably spread widely and could not be kept at bay with stop-and-go policies that would prove unacceptable in the long run. General lockdowns, they said, were last-resort measures that brought countries into uncharted territory, with many potentially adverse consequences, and it would become difficult to decide when and how to exit from this state of closure and to avoid flare-ups absent any reliable treatment (Sayers, 2020).

This position quickly attracted criticism in the scientific community and beyond, both at home and abroad. To many, it more or less amounted to letting the virus run free and waiting for some herd immunity. Although the Swedish authorities refrained from officially using this particular choice of words, it soon became clear that it was one of the expected side-effects of their mitigation strategy. However, hoping for such an immunity could be deemed somewhat in contradiction with the recommendation that people shield themselves from the virus as much as possible. In the UK, Prime Minister Boris Johnson had initially, and more openly, endorsed a strategy of achieving herd immunity, but had to back off quickly when an influential report from the Imperial College of London forecast skyrocketing mortality. In this respect, the Swedes were among the least impressed by the dire predictions of British epidemiologist Neil Ferguson that arguably contributed to the impressive spread of lockdown policies.

The Swedish approach – at first essentially based on recommendations, voluntary changes of behaviour and reciprocal trust to avoid closing society altogether – appears to some extent coherent with a Swedish system of crisis management based on openness, protection of civil rights and liberties and confidence in scientific expertise (Gras, 2020). However, the history of handling epidemiological risks shows that Sweden has a record of more stringent interventions, as in the case of AIDS (or cholera long before), and could rely on a communicable disease law to hold citizens responsible for spreading infection (Baldwin, 2021). Anders Tegnell himself was one of the actors behind the mass vaccination of Swedes to prevent an episode of swine flu in 2009 that did not materialize. In the COVID-19 crisis, conflicting representations of Sweden started to emerge that stressed the betrayal of basic human values in a welfare state that should protect all citizens and provide good care, especially to the frail elderly. Here, the central role of experts could be reconciled with two interpretations, seeing experts either as independent minds in the service of the common good, pragmatic spirits versed in evidenced-based science and policy, or as the representation of cold social engineering and lack of empathy in a world of liberalized welfare and health care services (Lundqvist and

Petersen, 2010). In this battle of interpretations, political and moral judgements were never far off, and Sweden became a case in point in the new and thriving business of comparing national strategies, their legitimacy and their efficiency on a nearly daily basis.

In truth, nowhere else in the world did one single public expert – namely Anders Tegnell – attract so much attention, fascination and also resentment during this crisis. (Anthony Fauci, the main scientific spokesman for the White House Coronavirus Task Force, probably came close, albeit under a president who was not ready to play second fiddle.) This is a highly unusual phenomenon for Sweden, where experts and bureaucrats rarely attract so much public attention. In 2020, the state epidemiologist became the subject of sheer fanaticism and hatred well beyond Sweden – almost on a par with environmental activist Greta Thunberg in recent years – to the point that his daughters auctioned five minutes of his 2020 Christmas evening to raise money for a charity. To some, he best embodied the Swedish way of doing things: pragmatic, no-nonsense, calm. But again, it was easy to see in him the opposite qualities of the cold social engineer, lacking compassion and blinded by his convictions.

The Swedish puzzle

Explaining this Swedish 'anomaly' in the Covid-19 crisis is not an easy task. Many have portrayed it as the result of a single strategy of 'herd immunity' that did not publicly say its name (Anderberg, 2021). If one European country went in this direction, it is most probably Sweden, but when specific tests started to reveal that only a fraction of the population had antibodies – before the summer of 2020 – Swedish experts must have been faced with the fact that natural immunity was not close at hand. However, although they admitted to some misjudgements and later failures, they did not radically modify their approach and recommendations, even during a second wave that proved equally lethal. The comparatively high degree of autonomy of Swedish public administration in relation to the political branch and the relative weakness of legal instruments – such as the lack of provisions for a state of emergency in peacetime – have ranked among the frequent arguments offered to account for this deviation (Jonung, 2020). They should not be overlooked and certainly played a role, even in the differentiation between Sweden and its direct Nordic neighbours. In Denmark, the government should have acted upon advice from the health agency, but the prime minister, Mette Frederiksen, quickly stepped in to have the existing legislation modified and give the government more power. In Sweden, the Parliament (Riksdagen) did vote on temporary extraordinary powers to the executive, in April 2020, so that it could shut down specific venues, but they were not used. Summertime provided a respite, and the weak signals of flare-up in the autumn strengthened the hope that the Swedish strategy had somehow paid off.

At the beginning of the second wave, in November 2020, the Swedish government appeared to be willing to play a stronger part and a bill was presented to the Riksdag to prepare for a new pandemic legislation that would take effect in January 2021. During all this time, of course, political actors were not passive, but their presence on the scene stood in sharp contrast with most other countries, where, for better or worse, politicians firmly took the reins. The political consensus remained high, with the exception of the growing national populist right-wing party, Sweden Democrats (SverigeDemokraterna [SD]), which voiced dissent, urged stricter measures and called for the resignation of the government. In fact, the COVID-19 crisis added to a difficult political situation in Sweden: since 2014, Social Democratic Party coalitions had depended on fragile agreements with the Centre-Right to insulate against the rising nationalist party.

If countries such as the UK, the US, Italy or France were facing a deep organizational crisis as a result of the pandemic, improvising policies and sending unclear or arbitrary messages to their populations (Bergeron et al, 2020), Sweden seemed at first to play it almost by the book, respecting the traditional division of responsibilities between state, administration and local government, relying on pandemic plans, on available scientific expertise and on WHO recommendations and using a communication style meant to deter panic and fear. The emphasis was on following recommendations, and the best way to achieve voluntary compliance was to give citizens the basic tools to act responsibly, to resist the wave of disinformation that burst out around the world and to foster a climate of reciprocal trust between people and institutions. To some extent, Sweden managed to achieve just this, which is in itself a rather remarkable result in a pandemic crisis that wreaked havoc everywhere. However, cracks started to show on the varnish: the experts and public authorities were accused early on of underestimating not only the risks but also the consequences in terms of mortality or saturation of hospitals; they were blamed for issuing recommendations based on weak or contradictory scientific evidence, i.e., when it came to wearing masks. Recommendations were also influenced by the lack of material supply or preparedness; politicians were criticized for hiding behind experts and bureaucrats while leaving citizens with the responsibility to adopt the proper conduct and limit the spread of the virus.

It is as though the Swedes somehow bound themselves to this particular mitigation strategy, convinced that its overall costs would be more acceptable in the long run and that lockdowns would most likely only postpone circulation of the virus, making it hard to decide when and how to open society again and bringing unforeseeable consequences. They were not entirely wrong in this prognosis, but they also anticipated that the virus would be easier to trace and less lethal and that vaccines would not arrive as fast as they did. Succeeding on this risky path implied protecting the most vulnerable, in the first place older people who needed personal assistance. With a limited supply of protective gear and hospital beds and a decentralized structure governing care, the recommendations of FHM to shield the frail elderly ran the risk of becoming empty words. Indeed, nearly half of the mortality in the first wave affected nursing homes and many people died without receiving appropriate medical care. In spite of strict lockdowns, France and even the UK did not fare better in this respect, but within the Nordic region, the Swedish performance does not look pretty at all. Sweden suffered a mortality ten times higher than Denmark, Finland and Norway during the first wave.

In this book, I will show that the distinctive Swedish path is quite coherent with Sweden's institutional framework and procedures designed for times of crisis and with the lack of specific legal instruments for peacetime emergencies. In this sense, it departs significantly from the situation in many other countries where emergency measures and special legislation were commonly used, making possible exceptional policies on a grand scale such as national lockdowns, curfews, border closings and other restrictions of civil liberties. However, even if the Swedish strategy can easily be reconciled with the basic tenets of crisis management and the significant autonomy of bureaucratic agencies or local government – which was repeatedly stressed by the main actors – it is still in contradiction with previous experiences of epidemic response in this country, which were characterized by stronger interventionism (Baldwin, 2021). In addition, the particular political context of a weak government and a prime minister who did not wish to be first on the front lines reinforced the traditional division of power in favour of the expert bureaucracy. It produced the exceptional situation in which a state epidemiologist – Tegnell – became the public face of Sweden and was seen to bear the brunt of responsibilities during the crisis. Andersson and Aylott aptly described this Swedish case as 'unexceptional exceptionalism' (Andersson and Aylott, 2020), which captures the paradox of a crisis management that apparently followed the standard procedures but was overwhelmed by the magnitude of the events, by their global scale and by the controversies that the Swedish line triggered.

The case of Sweden allows discussion of recent theorization of the pandemic response in terms of 'organizational crisis'. This type of approach rightly places the emphasis on problems of coordination and cooperation in societies otherwise saturated by organizations. It also considers that major crises instil political panic, leading to emergency responses that may deviate from standard operation plans, bypass the (democratic) circuits of responsibility and create ad hoc organizations that make coordination even harder. This can, in turn, lead to radical policy choices sometimes decided on the fly, such as national lockdowns (Bergeron et al, 2020). In the case of Sweden, however, we witnessed almost the exact opposite phenomenon, at least at face value: the authorities remained strangely calm all along – even under severe pressure to change course – and they followed the essential guidelines, mostly respected the power equilibrium and trusted their citizens to abide by recommendations; no emergency order was ushered in, as there is no such provision for peacetime, and policy changes remained comparatively incremental and moderate. However, this did not prevent Sweden from facing important coordination problems, and in this respect the country lacked strategic capacity at the government level (Ahlenius, 2020; Pierre, 2020). This study will not aim primarily to evaluate the Swedish record in terms of mortality and other impacts, but it can contribute to a better understanding of the entanglement that led Sweden down this unique pathway and of the intense controversies that it triggered.

Shifting representations of the Swedish model

Trying to account for the peculiarities of the Swedish response and evaluate their consequences is one thing, but it is also important to pay attention to the justifications that the actors themselves gave for their choices and to the intense controversies it triggered at home and abroad. All along, Anders Tegnell and FHM, in charge of the response, enjoyed approval rates above 60%; they only fell below this threshold for Tegnell at the end of the second wave in the spring of 2021. The government and prime minister enjoyed support of about 40%, but Stefan Löfven remained the most popular among party leaders. Hardly anyone was sacked or had to resign, with the exception of the head of the Civil Contingency Agency (Myndighet för samhällskydd och Beredskap, MSB), who was caught red-handed travelling for leisure in the winter of 2020. Nevertheless, a special commission of inquiry was set up as early as June 2020 and issued its first report the following autumn, pointing to a number of collective and institutional failings in the response to the crisis, with a particular emphasis on old-age care (Coronakommissionen, 2020).

Sweden did not fundamentally change tack, even though a series of stricter measures were enforced at the end of 2020 and temporary pandemic legislation was prepared in the context of mounting political pressure. A form of public health nationalism seems to have prevailed all along, one that left only limited space for internal criticism in the media. The level and tone of domestic controversies were nonetheless unusual for Sweden, and the national strategy received widespread attention abroad, affecting the traditional patterns of support for a Swedish model that feeds on foreign representations. Indeed, for almost a century, images of Sweden have revolved around the theme of continuous progress (Musial, 2002; Aucante, 2013a). Until recently, perhaps no other country in the world had so fully epitomized the values of welfare, redistribution, equality, and solidarity and the possibility of reconciling them with economic performance. This image started to waver in the 1990s in the wake of financial crisis, increased liberalization of the welfare system and rising inequalities (Ryner, 2002; Andersson, 2009b). Over time, the great conceptual flexibility embedded in this idea of a Swedish (or Nordic) model has lent itself to ongoing reinterpretations in the repertoire of social and economic progress (Cox, 2004). This 'swedophilia' suffered occasional blemishes when pamphlets vilified the 'new totalitarians' (Huntford, 1971) or mocked the 'almost nearly perfect people' (Booth, 2015) of northern Europe. The dominant storytelling has been one of success and adaptation to the challenges of a globalizing world for small countries that topped international rankings of all kinds. There has been, however, a long-term tendency to use the Swedish model as a flexible tool in political controversies, perhaps since US journalist Marquis Childs published his famous essay on 'The Middle Way' in 1936 (Childs, 1936).

Since that era, Sweden has also developed a powerful public diplomacy to bolster its favourable credentials abroad (Clerc and Glover, 2015), in spite of occasional conflicts such as with the US during the Vietnam War. In recent years, the country did not enjoy the same amount of sheer financial power that oil-rich Norway could deploy to support its reputation as a 'moral superpower', but it nevertheless managed to compensate thanks to an acquired symbolic capital as a principled player in international politics, and positioned the Swedish model as a successful 'brand' (Browning, 2007; Marklund, 2016).

One hypothesis is that the handling of the pandemic and its justifications fell into the pattern of Swedish exceptionalism while at the same time upsetting some basic components of what is regarded as the Swedish model and deeply affecting the image of Sweden not only abroad but also within the Nordic region. It is indeed striking to see that most explanations, justifications or criticisms of the Swedish anomaly have resorted to basic – and generally selective – elements of the model discourse. In many ways, it took the shape of a fierce symbolic and even normative battle – through online media and speeches or interviews to (re)define the meaning of the model and its coherence or conflict with the Swedish management of the crisis. As usual, there was also an evident hiatus between domestic debates, on the one hand, channelled through mainstream media and more or less constrained in their criticism of public policies, and foreign images, on the other hand, that appeared to be slightly more polarized. To some extent, it bore some resemblance to discussions surrounding the Icelandic financial and political crisis after 2008: in that case, the common and idealized representation – mediated by international rankings – of an Icelandic egalitarian democracy devoid of corruption shrivelled, especially in countries (such as the UK) that were direct victims of the Icelandic banks' collapse. At the same time, there was also a growing interest in what was regarded as democratic revival and experiments during the crisis, and the Icelandic elites shrewdly managed to sell the moral image of a small country fighting for survival (Chartier, 2011; Ingimundarson et al, 2016; Aucante and Aucante, 2017).

Sweden has much more international visibility than Iceland, but there are definitely parallels in the uses of the Nordic countries as democratic epitomes. However, what is strikingly different this time around is that the traditional patterns of support for a progressive Swedish model have been turned almost upside down. In spite of the gradual translation of social democracy towards the Centre-Right and of the liberalization of European welfare states, the vestiges of the model are still embraced as a thing of the Left synonymous with a reconciliation of social welfare and rights, public services and economic performance. To be sure, contemporary reforms in these fields have pulled in new fans from the neoliberal spectrum (Economist, 2013), and the rising national populists in Sweden have also tried to position themselves as defenders of a more chauvinistic welfare system. But the Swedish response to the pandemic led to dismay and criticism among most – not all – classical supporters of the model, while ideological families that are more prone to despise what Sweden stands for (e.g., libertarians or even national populists) shifted to hail the country as a defender of civil liberties. This probably came as a surprise in Sweden, where criticism of the strategy was indeed voiced but without a clear notion that it would ignite such a conflagration of controversies abroad. As a result, Swedes were perhaps eager to back up policy choices that left them some degree of freedom to act as they saw fit, and some observers believed that it reflected the unorthodox balance between statism and individualism so characteristic of Sweden (Trädgårdh, 2020; Tubilewicz, 2020).

A second hypothesis is that the pandemic put pressure on sections of the Swedish political and welfare system that have been under heavy strain for quite some time. As social reforms and public administration restructuring have been debated and implemented since the 1990s, they have gradually reshaped the health and care sector according to the doctrines of liberalization and new public management; unemployment protection is increasingly drifting away from universalism, and the influx of new migrants in recent years induce divisions and precariousness on the job market (Emmeneger et al, 2012; Berglund et al, 2020) while fuelling the nationalist discourse on a welfare and cultural crisis (Demker, 2014). The inroads of the nationalist Sweden Democrats Party have led to a situation of political instability with weak governments, and the COVID-19 crisis has in a way magnified all these trends as the 2022 elections are getting closer, emphasizing the question of political responsibility in a fragmented and decentralized regime. Given the magnitude of the crisis and the exposure of Sweden, COVID-19 has triggered a renewal of debate over policy options and will likely have an impact on political platforms for the 2022 election, although it is still unclear to what extent it can be a real game-changer. The moral implications of this crisis are indeed profound: they concern the construction and legitimacy of Sweden not only as a welfare state but also as a paragon of social progress in the larger Nordic region. To what extent was the pandemic response in blatant contradiction with what the Swedish model is supposed to stand for? Or should we rather conceive of the latter as an arena open to conflicting interpretations and ideological conceptions? I argue that the response was profoundly political and politicised, in the sense that it was used in a deeply ambiguous form of public health nationalism across countries that entailed trade-offs between civil liberties, the rule of Law, and a renewed concern for the collective protection of health.

The literature on this crisis has exploded across the span of the pandemic. Not only because many academics, intellectuals and journalists were stranded, but also because the intensity of the shock was rare, reshaping our daily lives in all sorts of ways, challenging a familiar organization of world affairs based on free trade, open borders, migrations and mass tourism. In addition, the sudden deluge of information and an explosion of social network activity produced a mass of data: statistics, analyses, opinions, fake news and conspiracy theories, mixing profane and expert contributions in a gigantic maelstrom. Comparisons of national cases and strategies, often with an implicit moral valuation, became the new normal. This study is based on the great variety of sources that have become available in these extraordinary times: (social) scientists not only wrote academic analyses, they also took positions in various medias, as did the author of these lines; statistics, science and expertise were the subject of intense debates at all levels; public agencies and decision makers gave press conferences and interviews on an almost daily basis and published data as well as other reports on their activities; governments launched special commissions to inquire into responsibilities during the crisis. All these materials constitute the backbone of this book.

Outline of the book

This book is about accounting for the Swedish deviation during the COVID-19 crisis, as well as about making sense of the intense controversies that it triggered at home and internationally in relation to changing representations of the Swedish model.

Chapter One deals with this highly flexible and ambivalent notion of 'model Sweden', tracing some of the intricate origins of discourses and representations of northern Europe, explaining the various dimensions that they came to incorporate, from social democracy and universal welfare to strong egalitarian norms but also specific forms of public administration and transparency. It also emphasizes some of the more recent changes and uses of this notion in light of social welfare and economic reforms that have taken place over the last three decades. The successful 'packaging' of these exemplary values through international diplomacy and branding strategies has been a trademark of the Nordics, and it reflects a unique capacity to produce a hegemonic narrative of progress, selecting dimensions that mostly confirm positive images and beliefs. It also functions as a permanent filter for (re)interpreting state and society even in the face of exceptional crises such as the 2020 pandemic. In this context, the controversies that appeared referred to different and potentially conflicting aspects of the model repertoire and impacted the common patterns of political support behind it. They also created a divide between the different Nordic countries, with Sweden as an outlier.

Chapter Two covers the outbreak of the epidemic and the specific responses of Swedish authorities during the first wave in the spring of 2020. It shows how the national strategy that diverged considerably from the rest of the North and of Europe is nonetheless quite coherent with conventional Swedish institutional arrangements and crisis management procedures: the strong autonomy of agencies and the authority of experts, the reliance on recommendations and discipline, the high level of decentralization for health-related matters as well as the lack of certain legal instruments. However, this response was also paradoxical in several ways and was met with great astonishment, especially in light of the fact that Sweden has one of the lowest hospital bed capacities in the OECD and that previous epidemics showed that it could act more forcefully. The responsibility of political decision makers was questioned, while the main controversy revolved around the issue of 'herd immunity' as an implicit strategy and the extraordinary role of a few experts in this respect. The combination of a particularly fragile political situation with this institutional fragmentation contributed to shape the Swedish deviation.

Chapter Three moves on to examine how the Swedish exception was perceived and why it became so hotly debated in light of international comparisons in spring 2020. Sweden has been more than ever in the spotlight. The daily briefings of Tegnell and his colleagues were followed by journalists and experts around the world. Initially there were more favourable opinions about a strategy that avoided lockdown and aimed to mitigate the overall effects of the pandemic, but it became increasingly controversial as the mortality rate deviated so much from the rest of the Nordic region. This chapter reflects on the comparison of policies, statistics, infection rates, death counts and the moral and normative dimensions that surrounded the justification of each nation's 'strategy'. It analyzes the nature and change of the discourses on the Swedish exception and their relationship to the trope of the Swedish model. In reaction to rising criticism of the Swedish line, a form of 'public health nationalism' emerged in Sweden. I show that this is coherent with traditional forms of trust in science, expertise and public institutions in this society but that it also hides a tendency to avoid divisions and conflicts. It may have positive aspects as well in times of crisis by creating a sense of stability and collective responsibility.

In Chapter Four, I examine the evolution of the epidemic response throughout the ensuing flare-ups. The slower resurgence of infections in autumn 2020 seemed to give some credit to the Swedish approach and resulted in a temporary return to international grace. Once again, Sweden became interesting and played a role in the debate over the use of lockdown strategies. While the experts still enjoyed a high level of trust, inquiries into the failure to protect vulnerable populations who lived in old-age residences or were dependent on home care services shed a negative light on crisis management and decision-making. The idea that democracy and political responsibility had been undermined by excessive trust in expertise and bureaucracy became more widely discussed, with a search for responsibility at different levels, but no witch hunt. The resurgence of the virus eventually led government and parliament to intervene more directly, devising a new pandemic law that was voted on in January 2021 and that opened for incremental restrictions, not always justified by new scientific evidence. The domestic debate on responsibility would continue throughout 2021 until the next report of the Coronakommissionen (Corona Commission).

Chapter Five presents conclusions about the changing representations of the Swedish model in relation to the handling of this pandemic crisis. There has never been so much focus on Sweden in a limited period of time. The model has for a long time been a source of interest around the world, attracting more positive views from the left of centre and more negative ones from the critics of egalitarian and redistributive policies. With ongoing public sector and welfare reforms since the 1990s, Sweden has gained new supporters from the economically liberal side. The hypothesis is that this crisis seems to have turned the classical lines of support upside down, with a new coalition of libertarians and populist right-wingers (except at home!) now more prone to praise the Swedish defence of civil liberties and of business interests and the responsibility of citizens to respect health recommendations, whereas traditional supporters have been more critical of the failure of an advanced welfare state to protect its vulnerable elderly population. However, the crisis raised important questions about the long-term impact of welfare, health and social care reforms, and particularly the organization of elderly care. In the first phase of the crisis, there was considerable interest in the international media about a 'strategy' that avoided lockdown and strict constraints. Then, as mortality rose, the misleading idea that Sweden did nothing to fight the virus and only waited for herd immunity did a lot of harm to the image of the country abroad. There was a mobilization to explain publicly and in diplomatic and international business circles that Sweden was not passive and should not be treated as a pariah state. By the end of 2020, the controversies had created problems even regionally, with tensions at the border between Norway and Sweden. Foreign discourses and images – with their biases – in this sense are not just symbolic; they affect a nation's place in world affairs and may also influence domestic policies and public diplomacy in return. Whether this impact will be temporary or persistent remains an open question.

ONE

The Uses of National Models

Scandinavia arguably stands out as the only region in the world to have been associated with a history of social, economic and democratic progress for over a century. Indeed, it has been relatively spared from the curse of war and authoritarianism. Among the three countries that make up this geopolitical ensemble, Sweden holds a special position in this political imagery of a progressive, social democratic northern periphery of Europe. Through the particular historical genealogy of the Nordic and Swedish models as paragons of progress, moral qualities of social justice and solidarity, humanitarianism, equality and civic-mindedness have been attributed to these countries (Musial, 2002; Aucante, 2013a). One of the important features of the Swedish model lies in its allegedly universal welfare system: social benefits are considered to be generous and all-encompassing, they are partly tax-financed and they enjoy high support in society (Rothstein, 1998). Starting from the guarantee of a minimum standard of living, this type of welfare regime has evolved to provide extended social services, social rights and a high level of redistribution. At one point in time, it went so far as to allocate certain social goods irrespective of work or professional status, as a form of 'decommodified' social protection (Esping-Andersen, 1990). However, high taxes and public spending have been the logical counterpart to finance this system. Therefore, the outstanding capacity of these small nations to reconcile economic performance and development with welfare and redistribution has also been key to their long-standing reputation as models.

Social democratic parties and closely associated labour unions have been another essential element of the Nordic welfare regimes. In Sweden, the Social Democratic Party has been in office for the greater part of the postwar era. For this reason, it is also a strong component of the modern political identity and image of the country, although its position is no longer as dominant as it used to be. For a long time, the party assumed the responsibility of governing alone, even when it had to rely on some degree of external support in parliament (Aucante, 2020a). Formal coalitions (with the Green Party, for instance) have now become more necessary and, since 2014, the Social Democratic cabinets headed by Stefan Löfven have been characterized by their precarious position and a dependence on painful agreements with Centre-Right parties. There have been continuous debates about the transformation of social democracy and of welfare regimes, the extent to which they have been substantially altered by neoliberalism and the programme to reform public services, possibly resulting in more inequality and less redistribution (Ryner, 2002; Pontusson, 2005). Sweden has been a case in point as the resilience of parties and policies on the Left have been tested in the context of globalization (Thelen, 2014). At the same time, the Swedish/Nordic capacity to adjust to these conditions of international competition and implement reforms deemed to foster the effectiveness and sustainability of public social spending has been considered an asset, although it could mean departing from the traditional social democratic model of welfare (Freeman et al, 2010).

Other important dimensions of the model relate to the functioning of democracy in the broadest sense and to the relation between state and society. The importance of social compromise between state, business and unions – but also between parties – has allowed for a significant reduction of conflict and greater cooperation and trust between actors, with consequences not only for the way capitalism and production work but also for democracy more generally. In the early 1980s, Elder et al defined consensual democracy as a low level of conflict, a high degree of concertation and a strong regime legitimacy (Elder et al, 1982). This is not to say that conflicts do not exist or have not increased. Indeed, the rise of anti-tax and then national-populist movements since the 1970s have resulted in a more polarized political scene in the North, with conflicts over immigration policy and multiculturalism, for instance (Widfeldt, 2018). Yet even if the traditional pillars of social and political compromise have eroded, they still support the foundations of society. Sweden is formally a centralized state, but it is important to consider some of its peculiarities: it features a strong tradition of administrative autonomy, which means that ministers do not have the authority to steer bureaucratic agencies as they see fit. In addition, local governments also enjoy considerable welfare responsibilities and the capacity to raise taxes. For a long time, a system of public commissions representing diversified sectors of society and politics took charge of preparing and anchoring public policies, fostering deliberation and trust (Trägårdh, 2007). These institutions have clearly lost ground, yet there are still some remains of this recent past, and such commissions can play a role in times of crisis either in anticipating potential reforms or through public inquiries to assess responsibilities.

The idea of national (social) models is by and large a construct of postwar comparative social sciences that has been successful to the point of becoming a trope in public discourse and imagination (Stråth, 2006). However, this discourse is often poorly defined. When people – even journalists or academics – refer to 'the Swedish model', the meaning is seldom crystal clear. There is a fundamental duality and ambivalence to this idea, in the sense that it can mean two different things that have increasingly tended to be confused. First, a model can refer to the particular socioeconomic and political choices that a given country adopts and that constitute its distinctive profile, partly reflecting its sociocultural identity. Sweden, for instance, has a more tax-financed and universal welfare system, yet in spite of this its unemployment insurance system is still organized on a voluntary basis with contributions from employees, an arrangement that dates back to the 1930s and was meant to secure the influence of trade unions. The second dimension is evaluative and normative and has to do with the comparative performance of models on the market, according to varying criteria. In this light, some models may be considered better than others and worth emulating. Indeed, most representations of the Swedish and Nordic models have been positively and normatively laden, as a synonym of continuous social, economic and political progress, which is a rather unique phenomenon. Political scientist Francis Fukuyama went so far as to coin the expression 'getting to Denmark' to capture his idea of an ideal democratic society in our contemporary world (Fukuyama, 2011). He was not much concerned with whether the Danish reality deviated from this ideal-typical model, arguing that Denmark came close enough to the constitutional and democratic norms that one could wish for.

The model discourse has been a construction made from outside in the first place, a form of 'xenostereotype', although it subsequently became a co-construction through the particular relationship that Scandinavia developed with the rest of the world (Bergman, 2007). For Sweden, the best historical example is probably the series of books American journalist Marquis W. Childs published in the 1930s with telling titles: *The Middle Way* and *This is Democracy* (Childs, 1936, 1938). The works had an enduring effect on the image of Sweden as a nation in the progressive vanguard, especially in the US, though there were also detractors of this 'swedomania' bordering on socialism (Kettunen and Petersen, 2022). With the postwar reconstruction and the East–West conflict, Sweden came to be seen as a 'middle way', a politics of conciliation between capitalism and socialism. The construction of this discourse continued and diversified during the 1960s and 1970s, when French journalist Jean-Jacques Servan-Schreiber probably coined the term 'Swedish model'

(Servan-Schreiber, 1968). There were also rare but notorious critiques, such as British journalist Roland Huntford's book *The New Totalitarians*, which ferociously stigmatized a Swedish progressive myth that hid more conformist and authoritarian tendencies (Huntford, 1971). More generally, the vision of Sweden fluctuated politically with respect to the national context of its production, in as much as it was meant to reflect on virtues that could be seen under the Northern Lights and were likely to be missing at home.

Swedes and their neighbours have certainly developed a particular sensitivity to all these foreign images of their own way of life, representing themselves through the looking glass. Their favourable reputation was also prolonged through their diplomatic efforts to appear as moral and humanitarian ambassadors on the international scene, particularly in the Global South (Nilsson, 1991; Clerc et al, 2015). From the 1980s on, the model discourse started to turn into a real smörgårsbord, to use a Swedish word borrowed by the English language. At a time when international rankings and benchmarking became the new game in town, the Nordics regularly flocked near the top places with respect to equality, well-being, transparency or freedom. In the era of neoliberal globalization, these small exporting countries suffering from the industrial crisis felt the pressure to diversify their economies and markets to bolster their competitive advantage. The new economic and managerial doctrines of the time had an impact on the Nordic social democratic regimes, not least in Sweden. They opened the way for substantial programmatic shifts and reforms of the state, of public services and of social benefits. Hence the model discourse ended up being conceptually stretched to incorporate the remarkable capacity of the Nordic states to adjust to the vicissitudes of globalization while still performing well in many areas (Cox, 2004). In this way, it risked running on empty.

For a very long time, Nordicity has been a valuable product on the global market of reputation, a kind of brand attached to a specific lifestyle and most famously translated into Scandinavian architecture and design (Browning, 2007). The contemporary wave of globalization has intensified the search for competitiveness with an increasing importance of soft power and new modes of communication. While the cost of social spending used to be a primary target of the neoliberal mantra, efficient and well-equipped welfare, health care and educational systems are now regarded as an asset for corporations and their multinational staff, who put a premium on good working and living conditions. Since 2020, the pandemic crisis has placed countries, and particularly welfare states, under unprecedented pressure to compare their overall performance and justify their choices in the name of protection against the new virus. Instead of the usual economic race, we have witnessed a form of health competition and even health nationalism, with Sweden playing the role of an outlier. In some respects, this is not completely new for a country that has been non-aligned for so long, although Swedes were not used to so much criticism. What has changed, however, is the pattern of foreign political support for a Swedish strategy hailed by a strange coalition of libertarians, neoconservatives and populists, whereas attitudes were politically reversed at home under a Social Democratic administration. Indeed, on the grounds of trust or discipline, many a Swede considered that the authorities were simply following the local precepts of good crisis management, in spite of mounting domestic criticism.

This first chapter does not intend to re-collect all the scattered pieces that have composed the Swedish model discourse over time, which would be a much too large ambition. The main goal is to better understand the representations behind it that can be mobilized and have been used selectively to explain, justify or criticize the Swedish strategy during this world crisis. Furthermore, the pandemic helps cast some light on the gaps between the traditionally positive images of Sweden and the less visible, more complex dimensions of this society that are nevertheless part of its national construction. The added strains the pandemic placed on welfare and care and the high death toll in Sweden compared to the other Nordic states may possibly give new energy to the long-standing debate over cycles of reforms that were meant to enhance both performance and profitability and may have increased the vulnerability of the system to crises such as the present one.

The contradictions of progressiveness

As Swedish historian Bo Stråth argues, 'memory and myth are mutually reinforcing entities' in the construction of national identities (Stråth, 2006, p 375). They are mixed together to produce narratives of the past. In the case of Sweden, progressiveness is a dominant narrative that incorporates many different ingredients such as individual and collective emancipation (from 'free' peasants to workers) leading to democracy, the development of universal welfare, a commitment to egalitarian values and more peaceful accommodation on the labour market. Progressiveness also rhymes with economic growth and technological innovation, solidarity with poor and oppressed countries, peace-building and, more recently, a high profile on environmental issues. Containment of class conflicts that once ran high in the early twentieth century was one of the main achievements of the social democratic movement and labour unions working closely with other parties and business interests. It laid the ground for the institutionalization of a particularly organized form of welfare capitalism that triggered considerable political and academic interest around the world (Castles, 1978; Esping-Andersen, 1985). Sweden and the other Nordic countries have increasingly been active in consolidating this credit and building on it through their strong engagement in international organizations and shrewd use of public diplomacy to promote their interests. Nordicity and Swedishness have become reputable brands, but it is important to recall that negative and downgrading representations of Sweden also abound, although they are less visible. To some extent, this flip side of the coin is an integral part of the ambivalence in the model discourse and of its political uses. In recent times, this dimension has grown more conspicuous, and the COVID-19 crisis reinforced that trend.

The dialectical nature of the Swedish model

According to Stråth again: 'The emerging patterns of social organisation merged hierarchy and centralized state authority with local community as the basis of government' as well as with 'an individual-oriented protestant responsibility and ethics' (Stråth, 2012, pp 29–30). Herein lies the unresolved tension between collectivism and individualism, equality and freedom that led historian Lars Trägårdh to coin the term 'statist-individualist' to describe modern Swedish political culture (Trägårdh, 1997). In Sweden, the strength of the state does not lie primarily in government, which is contained, but has to do with the role of the bureaucracy and public services and with the formidable expansion of the universal welfare system all the way to the local levels. Indeed, municipalities and regions have come to play a growing role in the provision of social services and care, although a large number of these services may be outsourced to private actors nowadays.

The Swedish political culture has also been portrayed as an entrenched democracy in which, for instance, the distance between the ruling elite and citizens is limited and transparency laws provide easy access to public proceedings and correspondence. Sweden boasts one of the oldest acts on press freedom, dating back to 1766. Journalists were thus able to investigate the actual strategy of FHM, the Swedish Public Health Agency, early on in the COVID-19 crisis. Institutions such as the Ombudsmän for Justice (which dates back to 1809), and the more recent Equality Ombudsman along with the Ombudsman for Children have also been influential innovations for the protection of civil rights, and any citizen can lodge complaints with these offices. They play an important role of judicial review. For instance, the chief ombudsman for justice expressed notable reservations with respect to the temporary pandemic legislation of 2021 and its prolongation.[1] Sweden was also one of the first states to start an independent commission of inquiry on public actions during the COVID-19 crisis, in June 2020.

The contradictions of the Swedish model are not something new, although arguably they have taken on a new dimension in the current crisis. The quest for social perfection through the faith in science, expertise, technocracy and social engineering has been a common theme in the understanding of Swedish society, leading to conflicting reinterpretations of the past, sometimes through the lens of contemporary values (Hirdman, 1989). This was the case for eugenics legislation in the 1930s, a widespread phenomenon at a time when racial biology was in the air. Over several decades, thousands of people – mostly women – were subjected to sterilization procedures because they were deemed unfit for reproduction on the basis of biased medical judgment (Broberg and Roll-Hansen, 1996). For a long time, the dominant conception of history emphasized peaceful accommodation between classes or interests and granted little attention to more or less violent deviations from this trajectory. Local historians and social scientists have made amends and started to uncover some of the less shining sides of the Swedish story, with its share of conflicts, oppression and discrimination (Andersson, 2009a). Foreign academics have perhaps not followed suit to the same extent, so that the Northern Star has continued to glow brighter from afar, at least until this pandemic. In this respect, critical viewpoints from abroad have become, for the most part, the responsibility of journalists or freelance intellectuals. It was quite common at the time when the Swedish economy was booming to find negative comments like Dwight D. Eisenhower's remarks at the 1960 Republican National Convention: the US president spoke of a European country where socialism had produced alarming rates of suicide and drunkenness. Although Eisenhower apologized for getting some of his facts wrong later, on the occasion of a visit to Sweden, the myth of a high suicide rate in Scandinavia persisted, as if it were the price to pay for a socialist type of welfare. A year later, British poet and critic Kathleen Nott, who resided for a while in Sweden, provocatively entitled her portrait of the country *A Clean, Well-Lighted Place*; the representation of conformism, discipline and hygiene that she gave stood in stark contrast with the reputation of moral and sexual liberty, or even depravity, commonly associated with Sweden and conveyed in films or literary works of this era (Nott, 1961). In the early 1970s, British press correspondent Roland Huntford lambasted the subservient, red-tape loving Swedes in his political essay *The New Totalitarians* at the very moment when the country was undergoing a profound cultural revolution as old forms of hierarchies and paternalism unravelled (Huntford, 1971; Marklund, 2009). It may also be appropriate here to quote German writer Hans–Magnus Ezensberger, who published travel diaries from various European countries in the 1980s and who also delivered a harsh judgment on Sweden's bureaucratic society. Indeed, his words strangely echo with the extraordinary trust that Swedes have placed in FHM and in its state epidemiologist, Anders Tegnell, during the pandemic: 'Whether it is ... about alcoholism, urban planning or health care, about the upbringing of their children or the taxation of their salaries, the citizens of Sweden are always willing to meet their authorities faithfully and trustingly, as if their benevolent disposition would be beyond any doubt' (Ezensberger, 1982, my translation).

As we can see, even though the motif of progressiveness and uniqueness of Sweden may be dominant, it has often existed in close interaction with other, more complex or negative themes that sometimes make Sweden appear almost a dystopia or an 'anti–model' (Aucante, 2013b). This is an important nuance to analyses that insist on the overwhelmingly positive imagery of Sweden and Scandinavia as a northern utopia, as there seems to be a fundamentally dialectical construction of the Swedish model discourse in the long run. The role Sweden played in comparisons of national strategies to battle COVID-19 is a rather fascinating illustration of this dialectical tension that conveys normative, even moral undertones. Journalist Paul Rapacioli, the founder of digital news network The Local has documented how contemporary media and politicians have increasingly abused this 'good Sweden/bad Sweden' ambivalence in recent years, circulating fake news, distorting reality or pulling selected facts out of context to show that Swedish society was very different from what it is believed to be, and certainly far from ideal (Rapacioli, 2018b). The focus has been mostly on immigration, crime and the far Right, and it seems that the wave of immigration in Europe in 2015 was a turning point in this respect (Truedsson, 2018). At first glance, this attention to negative images of Sweden is most visible in US, British and perhaps Russian media and much less so in the rest of Europe, yet social media now transcend borders and spread news, fake or not, at lightning speed in the era of post-truth. Rapacioli shows how Swedish examples were picked up and often twisted throughout the Brexit debate on immigration and also in the Trump campaign and presidency in relation to similar topics, as evidenced by the viral effect of Trump's speech about what happened 'last night in Sweden'[2] (Rapacioli, 2018a, p 87). All of a sudden, Sweden seemed plagued by violent crime, gangs and illegal immigration. Women would not dare to go out alone at night for fear of being raped. If it could happen in Sweden, the reasoning was, then no other country was safe from this civilizational threat. Perhaps all the criminal novels and TV series created by contemporary Swedish authors and producers and depicting a bleak Nordic world bear some responsibility for this new state of mind. After all, 'alternative facts' such as the ghetto-Sweden image are also a form of fiction, a creative distortion of reality, even if deprived and segregated urban areas do exist and violence can happen. Stieg Larsson, author of the renowned

Millennium trilogy, was himself a journalist and founder of the *Expo* journal that was committed to studying and fighting neofascist movements. Larsson's novels depict a deeply corrupt and schizophrenic Sweden, hiding all its violence under the veneer of a respectable society. In addition, the MeToo movement that began in 2017 and its deep repercussions in Sweden, a country known for its comparatively high degree of gender equality and consciousness, also conveyed the image of a more polarized country that did not always live up to its reputation.

The political and media offensive on the Swedish COVID-19 strategy may be seen in this particular context, but with one notable change: the kind of parties and ideologists who used to assert how bad Sweden had become in recent years, the same ones who remained sceptical of its welfare policies and its nanny state, were now among the first in line to praise the country for its defence of freedom, civil rights and business interests. Although part of the political Right has sometimes lauded Sweden's capacity to reform welfare for the sake of competitiveness, this was quite an unexpected reversal, particularly for a Swedish government led by the Social Democratic and Green parties.

From public diplomacy to Nordic branding

Swedish public institutions, media and interest groups have not only responded to the images and discourses about their country produced abroad, but have also helped to shape them in many ways. Sweden is endowed with formidable instruments of public diplomacy for a nation of its size. For example, the Nobel Institution that has granted prizes every year since 1901 for achievements in science, literature and peace not only provides visibility but also a form of superior moral authority and prestige. Ironically, the weapon magnate Alfred Nobel, who donated his fortune to the foundation, wanted the most important prize attributed to the Norwegian parliament, at a time when Norway was seeking full national autonomy after breaking away from the dynastic union with Sweden that had lasted since 1814. Nonetheless, as part of the Nobel Academy, the peace prize also indirectly affects the influence and reputation of Sweden in international affairs.

Studies have shown that 'Nordic governments and opinion-formers have not only been captives of, but also captivated by, their own national image abroad, which they have made long-standing attempts to curate and promote among foreign observers' (Clerc and Glover, 2015, p 7). This image and all the soft power associated with it have also been powerful instruments for the promotion of domestic economic and commercial interests abroad. The notion that social democratic welfare capitalism was a unique formula for success that could be exported had a great deal of influence from the 1930s on. As Carl Marklund has it, the welfare state has proven to be 'Scandinavia's best brand' (Marklund, 2016). At the turn of the 1960s, representatives of the Swedish business community and of trade unions toured jointly in places like the US to promote the spirit of negotiation and compromise that reigned in Sweden. Ironically, the 1960s were also a time of intense social unrest and wildcat strikes in Sweden. The early Swedish support in the United Nations for some colonized countries reclaiming self-determination, like Algeria in 1959, paved the way for solidarity with nations of the Global South, development aid and humanitarian assistance whereas ethnic minorities at home did not fare so well. Mobilizations against apartheid and to welcome refugees from South Africa also reached a turning point in the early 1960s (Sellström, 1999). The Swedish Institute, in charge of disseminating information about Sweden after 1945, linked diplomacy, culture and business and boosted the visibility of Sweden abroad. But other initiatives were taken in the early 1960s to promote Sweden's positive image internationally, such as the information collegium in charge of coordinating actors in the different fields of foreign affairs, culture, tourism and business.

From then on, official information on Sweden became more carefully and professionally monitored, even tailored to other countries' specific profiles: in other words, it was more relevant to emphasize democratic socialism for Africa and to put on a more business-friendly face in the US (Glover, 2015, pp 126–127). Interestingly, Nikolas Glover recalls discussions in the early 1970s about how to deal with some contentious and less attractive topics, for instance the depressing functionalist architecture of newly erected neighbourhoods of Stockholm such as Tensta (Glover, 2015, p 140). Fifty years later, this issue was still part of the debate on COVID-19 as the first clusters in spring 2020 were identified in these segregated urban areas, especially among Somali minorities, and the epidemic hit these communities much harder. At the time, Christian Democratic leader Ebba Busch tried to blame migrants for not learning enough Swedish language and culture to understand and apply health recommendations and was criticized in return for minimizing the role of socioeconomic inequalities or the type of professional activities that people in these neighbourhoods tend to take on (Busch, 2020).

Christopher Browning identifies two essential dimensions of Nordic branding, namely uniqueness and the fact that their model of society could be better and therefore worth studying and copying (Browning, 2007). The problem in the COVID-19 crisis was that the Nordic countries went separate ways, with Sweden going on its own. This deviation was heavily contested as unwise, even irresponsible, while Swedish authorities themselves considered their approach to be coherent with their institutional system and values. The relatively small countries of northern Europe have had a disproportionate influence and visibility in world affairs, which is in part due to their lasting reputation as a progressive vanguard, to instruments of public diplomacy and to their strong and relentless international engagement in multilateral institutions. But historical accidents have also had extraordinary global repercussions. For instance, this was the case with the 2005

Danish caricatures of the prophet of Islam, Mohammad, by the newspaper *Jyllands-Posten*, which triggered waves of protest throughout the Muslim world and had significant consequences for the position of Denmark abroad. The Icelandic financial and political crisis after 2008 is another recent illustration of this phenomenon: when the huge speculative banking system collapsed, it threatened not only the small island nation but also the assets of many foreign investors, particularly in the UK. The Icelandic crash and the political upheavals that followed received unprecedented international attention and revealed contrasting interpretations of the crisis and its impact, while Icelanders engaged in a lengthy and painful process to come to terms with this sudden financial craze (Ingimundarson et al, 2016; Aucante and Aucante, 2017). I believe the Swedish COVID-19 controversies fall somewhere in the same storyline and mobilize similar themes, such as the small-state resilience in adverse circumstances, the idea of exceptionalism and the peculiarities of Swedish democracy and values. These controversies also place an emphasis on important domestic debates, such as immigration and multiculturalism in the case of the Danish cartoons, crony capitalism in its Icelandic version or the neoliberal reforms and decentralization of welfare and care and the role of technocracy in Sweden. Finally, they appeal to a sense of national identity and even nationalism in spite of sharp divisions on home ground.

These particular crises show that each country in the region does not necessarily conform to a canonical Nordic model and that there is still room for significant divergences. The pandemic has left Sweden isolated and at some points blacklisted, an unprecedented phenomenon in itself. On both sides of the borders with its neighbours there was a great deal of incomprehension and even hard feelings in a region that is highly integrated and where free movement has been the rule since the mid-1950s, despite the fact that Norway is not a member of the European Union. The crisis also stirred up a form of rivalry on the terrain of welfare and good governance beyond what is commonly done in branding and ranking nations according to their indexes of performance in different areas. In fact, this rivalry has been coloured by moral overtones because of the higher death toll in Sweden.

Institutional dimensions of the Swedish model

The COVID-19 crisis has placed emphasis on many important dimensions of welfare and care as well as on the expanded role that the state has assumed – not everywhere and equally – to buffer the impact of the shock and compensate for some of the effects of the policies that reduced economic activities on a grand scale. This state expansion also moves in the direction of exceptional powers and means of control in the name of protecting populations. On these counts, the pandemic highlighted dilemmas and vulnerabilities that Sweden has faced in its reform trajectory; it also conferred a special yet ambivalent visibility to the Swedish model in relation to the larger question of democratic principles and governance.

Swedish welfare and care dilemmas in light of the pandemic

For the last three decades at least, Sweden has been at the centre of an intellectual and political debate about the nature and extent of welfare reforms. With the ideological shifts on the Swedish political scene since the 1980s and the deep financial and economic crisis of the 1990s came a wave of structural reforms that have deeply affected not only the welfare state but also the entire governance system. Sweden is arguably the Nordic country where these reforms have gone the furthest, but neighbouring nations have experienced similar trends.[3] In the process, the idea of a Swedish – or Nordic – model evolved in a way that is not unproblematic. As Robert Cox argues, there has always been a high degree of conceptual flexibility in this notion, encompassing different and new dimensions over time. It could eventually result in fuzziness or even tautology (Cox, 2004). But Cox himself adopts a definition of the contours of the model that lends itself to discussion, emphasizing the three dimensions of universality, solidarity and decommodification (that is, the degree of freedom from the market). As he rightly points out, these are already very broad sets of values, yet it is undeniable that the idea of a model transcends academic boundaries and has been widely used in the media and public discourse as well. As such, it is not a notion that is easily reducible to a few clear-cut dimensions. Not only have the contents changed over time, but academics have also contributed to this conceptual stretching more than they would like to admit.

Beyond this epistemological problem, what happened from the 1990s onward was a gradual transformation of the ideological position of the Swedish model along with the reforms that were justified on the grounds of the financial sustainability of the welfare system and also of the country's competitiveness. Hence the conjunction of reorganization and retrenchment, symbolized by the ambitious pension reform in the 1990s, progressively repositioned the Swedish model as a successful formula of adjustment to contemporary global capitalism that could appeal to the Right as well. Fredrik Reinfeldt's political offensive to recapture the model discourse and his close contacts with both New Labour and the Conservatives in the UK during his terms as Swedish prime minister from 2006 to 2014 were good evidence of these changes.

The point is not so much to judge whether Swedish welfare has changed beyond recognition, or changed for better or worse. This debate has almost endlessly mobilized intellectuals across disciplines and ideologies, and let us honestly say that the jury remains out. Some see the reforms as a way to enhance the efficiency and sustainability of public and social services while giving more freedom of choice to users. According to this view, Sweden has consistently featured among the top ten in the global economic competitiveness rankings of the World

Economic Forum, which also include criteria such as good health and education. Social spending decreased in the 1990s from about 30% to remain in the vicinity of 27%, on a par with its Nordic neighbours and much higher than the OECD average. In parallel, the development of universal childcare and more equal parental leave schemes has been regarded as a positive dynamic of social investment (Morel et al, 2011). Public funding of essential welfare and care services is still comparatively high as well, and social benefits are generous, although average pension and unemployment replacement rates have fallen considerably. For an average worker, net public pension rates fell from circa 85% in 1990 to just above 50% in 2015, which is now below the OECD average (Nelson, 2017).[4] Taking stock of this latter tendency, other scholars consider that Swedish welfare has undergone a significant overhaul, including a radical change in its philosophy (Andersson, 2009b). In this respect, social democracy is no longer the keeper of the sacred cow but has become one of the facilitators of systemic reforms (Klitgaard, 2007). Not only have income inequalities risen significantly, but private actors and insurance schemes have also made substantial inroads through the contracting out of public services and through insurance schemes intended to compensate for declining public benefits. Thus, marketization and managerial tendencies have pervaded most of the welfare system in the name of efficiency and freedom of choice. And, as Sweden continued to welcome immigrants more readily than its neighbours, classical universalism has increasingly come under strain: first, it fuelled socioeconomic inequalities; second, eligibility criteria and access to certain social benefits have been tightened; third, chauvinistic tendencies have developed at a quick pace, reclaiming a form of welfare based on more ethnic – or at least national – grounds. As Vanessa Barker argues, the result may be a new 'walling of the welfare state' that accentuates the repression of migrants (Barker, 2018).

The COVID-19 pandemic hit hard a number of sectors that have been reformed and could be more vulnerable. First among these are hospitals, which have been a target for rationalization and prioritization of ambulatory care, leading to a large-scale reduction of the number of beds since the 1990s. Management by performance triggered a movement of concentration toward bigger, more specialized institutions. Additionally, private corporations made inroads into health care. Conservative reformers of the National Health Service (NHS) in the UK even seemed to take a cue from the Swedish reforms in the 2010s that gave more freedom to private providers to distribute health centres on the basis of profitability rather than proven need and despite tax-financing (Ramesh, 2012). When COVID-19 hit the Stockholm area, some public hospitals could not count as much on their privately run counterparts to send staff over as they carried on with their daily routine of less urgent knee surgery or even cosmetic surgery. For example, the Södertälje Hospital west of Stockholm had to hastily recruit untrained staff to perform life-saving work (Erlandsson and Eriksson, 2020). With the pandemic, the just-in-time philosophy for supply and staffing and the fast-track patient discharge promoted in Sweden to reduce waiting times and raise profitability hit the wall. For this reason and in the context of an unknown virus, local governments and providers had to improvise constantly in the hard-hit areas and cope with a lack of essential materials. It will be important to evaluate and address the consequences of the enormous pressure that professionals have endured for months and will continue to bear due to the considerable backlog. Indeed, both difficulties in recruiting medical staff and long waits are likely to get worse in the wake of the pandemic. Actors in the field, such as the physicians' union, have pushed for a reform agenda with more state regulation and investment to deal with this backlog, which predated the pandemic.

The next sector that took a hard blow is elderly care. Sweden is an ageing country with 20% of its population 65 or older and one of the longest life expectancies on earth. Elderly care, once a cornerstone of public welfare, has been a prime target for competitive tendering since the 1990s, with about 20% of nursing homes contracted out, mostly to for-profit providers. Therefore, quality of care and local government capacity to monitor contracts have been regularly questioned (Blomqvist and Winblad, 2020). Today, residential and home care sectors rank among the largest employers in the country; the work conditions are difficult, and contracts are often precarious, forcing many employees – overwhelmingly women – to accomplish strenuous shifts in multiple nursing homes. In addition, there is a dearth of basic medical competence in Swedish elderly care, and municipalities are not even allowed to recruit medical staff directly. They are dependent on coordination with the regional level that is responsible for health care. This situation caused many elderly patients to be left without proper medical evaluation during the pandemic and to be prescribed palliative comfort care when their condition deteriorated.

In both sectors, health and elderly care, there are consequently notable departures from the classical picture of Swedish publicly funded universalism. As we will see, the state has not been passive, and public investment remains comparatively significant, but the locus of responsibility is decentralized, with many actors, and accountability is a problem. The strength of union organizations – such as Kommunal, which represents municipal service employees, or the unions of nurses and physicians – still provides checks and balances as well as coordination in a context of liberalization and flexibilization of the care sectors. This resilience of unions is one of the key factors emphasized by Kathleen Thelen in her comparative analysis of contemporary varieties of liberalization to show that Nordic social democracy still remains different (Thelen, 2014). However, it is not clear to what extent the pandemic will impact the dominant parameters of welfare and care organization in a country where new public management and private tendering is now so well entrenched. Because 2022 is an electoral year, with a change of prime minister and of

Social Democratic Party leader already in November 2021, the political implications of the pandemic are more likely to be part of the game. There are other points of vulnerability in Swedish welfare society that would certainly warrant discussion in relation to the pandemic and should at least be mentioned here. Voluntary unemployment insurance has many gaps, and youth unemployment is a problem. The condition of migrant communities is another important issue that has stirred debates. These populations were not only more at risk and more affected by the virus but also more likely to suffer economically. According to Statistics Sweden, unemployment among the foreign-born increased from 15.1% to 18.8% in 2020 as compared to a rise from only 5.1% to 5.8% among the Swedish-born.[5] However, the chauvinistic rhetoric of the increasing burden and risks that immigration poses to a Swedish model based on welfare and trust has been somewhat toned down during the crisis, with a few exceptions.

'Pandemocracy'

The global crisis that has been unfolding since 2020 has produced a surge of contradictory analyses and prognoses as to the nature of the shock that is proceeding before our eyes and, particularly, of its political implications. Scientific knowledge and expertise in times of uncertainty have been the subject of intense controversies, and conspiracy theories of all kinds that already had taken hold through social media have found the perfect climate to blossom and spread. In most countries, state intervention has been strong and has taken new forms, in particular through the use of universal lockdown of populations with the objectives of limiting or suppressing circulation of the virus and of averting complete saturation of hospitals. States of emergency were declared, and special legislation, powers and techniques of surveillance or quarantine were put in place, thus restricting a number of basic freedoms and rights in the name of protecting health and saving lives. National borders were shut down, bringing global trade and travel to a halt, although financial markets continued to function. Public debt and spending ceased to be a central problem, at least for a number of states that had good access to credit and were ready to open the floodgates in order to limit the harm to their economy and society. Paradoxically, the reinforcement of the state – in line with some of the tendencies identified in the post–Cold War neoliberal era (King and Le Galès, 2017) – was also a testimony to its structural weaknesses and policy incapacity in the face of the virus in many parts of the democratic world, whereas authoritarian regimes such as China displayed the full range of their disciplinary ability. Some regional organizations, such as the European Union, and international ones, particularly the WHO, managed to carve out a role for themselves in this highly nationalistic configuration.

In this extraordinary situation, Sweden has played an intriguing role as an outlier, resorting to an array of recommendations and relatively mild restrictions, shunning lockdowns and mask mandates and following a roadmap that did not substantially reinforce political leadership but rather gave pre-eminence to FHM and its bureaucratic experts while trusting the population to follow their recommendations. Because of the high death toll in comparison to its direct neighbours, the Swedish strategy has met with mixed feelings – especially from abroad – yet a majority of the local population seems to have supported this approach, with some inevitable ups and downs. Although there were controversies about the real intentions of FHM in relation to herd immunity and testing, as we will see, the degree of openness and transparency was higher than in many other places, with daily media briefings by the main agencies, countless interviews of Anders Tegnell and the early possibility to inquire about what was done. Access to the correspondence of participants, the nomination of a special 'corona' commission as early as June 2020 and other typical forms of judicial and administrative review contributed to the continuity of a democratic process that was also based on the participation and responsibility of citizens (Götz and Marklund, 2015). Parliament was reduced to 50 sitting members, but, because of the weak base of the Löfven cabinet, its prerogatives themselves were not reduced. In spite of the degree of consensus that prevailed, other parties did voice criticism or dissent and contributed to a new pandemic legislation, although belatedly. One could legitimately ask whether the respect for established procedures and division of responsibilities was not too high in a crisis that required a more diligent and forceful response, as in Denmark and Norway. Was it not necessary to better coordinate and oversee the local governments that are responsible for the bulk of the health and social care system? Or perhaps democracy was somewhat sidelined by a form of less accountable bureaucratic expertise that took on disproportionate importance given the uncertainty of the situation.

However, responding to a crisis of this magnitude is not just a question of institutional capabilities and material resources, which were lacking almost everywhere, even though countries that had previously been exposed to similar risks were arguably better prepared (Capano et al, 2020). Epidemic response is generally a complex balancing act that must rely on securing the compliance and support of the population over time. The paradox of the Swedish approach in the pandemic was that, while upholding a number of principles that traditionally make it stand out as a democratic model, it appeared to be contravening other important values such as the guarantee of universal access to good health care and the protection of basic welfare, in particular for the frail elderly. Although Swedish mortality rates remain lower than in many other European countries, the fact that they are still substantially higher than in the other Nordic nations that reacted earlier and more strongly casts an existential doubt on the Swedish line. More than ever, the pandemic underlines the fundamental ambivalences of the Swedish model construct and representations.

TWO

The First Wave

Between January and March 2020, the COVID-19 epidemic broke out in Europe and around the world. There are still many unanswered questions about the origin of the virus, the timing of its appearance and progression, and why some countries or regions, like northern Italy, were so rapidly and unexpectedly overwhelmed while others seemed to be relatively or entirely spared, at least during the first wave. In retrospect, at least three elements stand out in an otherwise still blurred picture:

1. Because the virus led to a high number of asymptomatic cases, it circulated under cover and had been around for some time when it was discovered.
2. The Western world and particularly Western Europe were hit much harder and earlier than other regions (apart from China) during this first sequence, but these countries had not been exposed to an epidemic risk of this magnitude and brutality for quite some time.
3. Even though each country had specific pandemic plans and preparations, heavily constraining lockdown policies rapidly became a standard response throughout Europe, with some variation in intensity.

Other parts of the world moved into the state of pandemic at different paces and with various strategies to adjust to the new threat. Yet the sum of all the national policies and the clear lack of coordination also contributed to the overall impact of the pandemic (Greer et al, 2020). Closing borders, shutting down airports, and cloistering people at home provoked a cascade of consequences of a magnitude rarely seen in modern times. In his book *Fighting the First Wave*, historian Peter Baldwin identified three broad families of countries according to the way they responded to the virus: 'targeted quarantiners' strictly tested, traced and isolated the sick; the 'ostrich family' favoured a hands-off approach; and another group of countries (potentially the largest) went into some form of national lockdown (Baldwin, 2021, p 4). There is obviously much more to this situation than meets the eye, as some countries were spared during the first wave or had histories of epidemic and other risks that made them more accustomed to extraordinary circumstances of this sort. Indeed, demography, the price attached to human life and the relationship to vulnerability or death vary greatly across the world.

Sweden is one example of a significant and possibly unexpected deviation, not only in the European context but among the advanced welfare states. Its official policy of mitigation was soon suspected to hide a search for some kind of herd immunity; its rebuttal of strict lockdowns, closures or even mask mandates, and its reliance on expert recommendations instead of political takeover, all stood in sharp contrast to other nation-states, even to its closest Nordic neighbours. In the apparent trade-off between freedom and security, it looked as if Sweden had gone for freedom first and was ready to pay any price upfront. As such, it was bound to attract attention because of the special role and image Sweden has enjoyed in world politics. Nevertheless, this does not imply that what was done there cannot be accounted for or amounts to a simple historical accident. It may appear paradoxical in light of the typical reaction of Swedish authorities to previous epidemic risks or episodes, such as AIDS, swine flu, and also cholera a long time ago (Baldwin, 2021). In each of those cases, the response was not so liberal or relaxed, and strict regulations and recommendations were issued, relying on a communicable disease law that formally allowed for registration and tracing while the penal code made citizens liable for purposely spreading infection (Christiansen et al, 2008).

In fact, part of the explanation of the Swedish approach must be grounded in Sweden's past experiences of facing such epidemic risks and other crises. The explanation is also inevitably multifactorial. The complex interplay of specific actors and institutions in a context of high uncertainty has already been the subject of some Swedish analyses that rely on unique access to communications made by public agents in the course of their duty. Johannes Anderberg's book *The Herd* (*Flocken*, 2021) is one such account. With a luxuriance of personal details, it follows the connections within the community of experts, epidemiologists, virologists and statisticians in Sweden and elsewhere, shedding light on the intricate choices, hypotheses and arbitrations that were made in the very first stages of the epidemic. Many other sources – such as daily briefings by Swedish authorities and intensive press coverage of them, interviews with the main actors, reports of various public commissions and parliamentary minutes – can contribute to the reconstruction and understanding of the decision-making process and to understanding public action in times of crisis.

Contrary to a widespread image conveyed in spring 2020, Swedish authorities did not remain utterly passive, even though they reacted sluggishly (Coronakomissionen, 2021). They made conscious choices based on available information and lessons from the past that were mediated by pandemic plans and a division of work between the political sphere and expert bureaucracy. Although they faced constraints, among them the lack of some strategic material (as almost everywhere else), they also had the resources with which to act differently than they did. They could have advised ski resorts to close earlier, recommended remote education for all levels, pushed for tighter controls on elderly care services or tried to pass special legislation with more haste as some Nordic neighbours did. They might have implemented a more stringent testing policy earlier on as well, especially to track asymptomatic cases. Alternative courses were indeed investigated and discussed among experts, and disagreements were voiced within the tightly knit community of experts surveilling this new virus. However, if the hope for herd immunity that proved so controversial was the ultimate goal, why did the Swedes persist so long in their approach once that hope faded and the prospect of vaccines came closer? They made a number of adjustments throughout the winter of 2020 and in the spring, but they did not so fundamentally change their line of conduct even as mortality kept rising and the authorities came under heavy pressure. The answer to this question must rely on an analysis of the sequence of events and of the various actors in the crisis.

The objective of this chapter is not to try to put together all the pieces of a highly complex jigsaw puzzle but rather to submit a set of hypotheses to the test and grapple with at least one central paradox: although the Swedish response was coherent in many ways with standard expectations in times of crisis, it was nonetheless considered exceptional, even unacceptable, to some – mostly foreign – observers. The case challenges or nuances an array of conventional ideas on the likely effects of public health crises, particularly that the central state and government usually prevail through emergency procedures in extraordinary circumstances (Bergeron and Castel, 2018). In the case of Sweden, in contrast, we witnessed a situation that was sometimes deemed an abdication of government (Ahlenius, 2020) but that more prosaically left important autonomy to expert bureaucrats, to local government and eventually to citizens, according to the constitution and the guiding principles of crisis management. At the same time, the Swedish approach also reflected both the concentration of responsibilities within a newly remodelled FHM and the dissemination of relevant scientific expertise among Swedish universities that went along with it (Anderberg, 2021). In other words, the agency was more influential but also less well equipped to confront crises of this nature. Finally, the government's resources for a stronger role had become limited as a consequence of previous crises, and it was also enfeebled by a political stalemate in effect since 2014, when elections did not produce clear parliamentary majorities. Thus, there was a combination of political and institutional (in)capacities and learning from past epidemic crises in a situation of uncertainty (Capano et al, 2020) but also a surprisingly limited coordination within the strongly integrated Nordic region.

Setting the stage

The new coronavirus spreading in China was already raising concern in Sweden by the end of January 2020. Early in February, it was deemed a significant risk by FHM, thus activating the crisis response process. The first case was detected on 31 January 2020; there were only seven official cases by the end of February. Hence the authorities considered circulation of the virus low, but at the same time many Swedes were returning from a number of Alpine ski resorts. Travellers were not systematically tested and were advised to return to work unless they had visible symptoms. Meanwhile, some countries such as Taiwan had already advised against travelling abroad, tightened airport controls and quarantines and banned exports of strategic materials during the last week of January (Anderberg, 2021). In east Asia the memory of Severe Acute Respiratory Syndrome (SARS) in 2003, although it was not associated with high mortality, had made countries more aware of the need to prepare for the next serious epidemic surge. The 2009 swine flu episode had also had a somewhat stronger impact in Asia. If the Swedish authorities did not react as strongly in February, this was on a par with other European countries where the circulation of the virus still seemed very limited. Some Swedish citizens were indeed repatriated from China and travelling there was not advised, but the risk of spread to the general population was considered low. However, the assessment was slightly different on the ground, in hospitals, as early as February, with some preparation already underway to withstand an epidemic surge (Löfgren, 2020).

Some Swedish experts, such as Björn Olsen, an infectious disease specialist known for a book on pandemics of this kind, had warned as early as mid-January that this one could be very serious and that Sweden was not necessarily well prepared as far as pandemic plans and equipment were concerned (Blume, 2020). It is a well-known fact that Sweden, along with Denmark, the UK and Mexico, has one of the lowest numbers of hospital beds in the OECD in proportion to its population, measured at less than 2.5 per 1,000 inhabitants in 2019, when France had nearly 6, Germany 8 and Japan 13.[1] This was equally true of intensive care beds, which also had been slashed, although not to the same extent. As I mentioned in Chapter One, the Swedish health care system went through deep reforms beginning in the 1990s and moved at a quick pace toward ambulatory care, limiting the duration of stays in hospital. In the 2018 election, health care was still hotly debated, particularly long waiting times for consultations and treatment and endemic shortage of staff (Holt, 2018). This low capacity should have been another reason for Sweden to be extra cautious about a new virus that might rapidly exhaust resources. Strangely enough, the situation of hospitals and their staffs did not make the headlines in Sweden as much as in countries such as France or the UK, where it became a crucial political indicator and a key pressure point for decision makers. Sweden may have failed in several respects, but hospitals nevertheless succeeded in reorganizing as well as they could in spite of capacities stretched very thin. However, it also implied stringent prioritization among older patients in hard-hit regions such as greater Stockholm (Savage, 2020).

Several factors can help explain the markedly different pandemic response in Sweden:

- There is a rather unique division of work between administrative and expert agencies, on the one hand, and the political decisional structure, on the other hand. In Scandinavia – but particularly in Sweden – public administrations enjoy a high degree of autonomy even in times of national crisis, and the Swedish constitution advises against ministerial steering (Jonung, 2020), even though there are other indirect forms of influence. In other words, public agencies are semi-autonomous and the constitution allows them to interpret the law and government directives. This regime is commonly criticized for limiting democratic accountability. In every country, bureaucrats obviously play a key role in times of crisis, but politicians are usually in the spotlight, for better or worse. Scientific experts naturally became more visible, but in Sweden it was FHM and its state epidemiologist Anders Tegnell – along with his team – who almost monopolized the front lines while the political elite appeared somewhat relegated to the background. Two other administrative units were key actors, namely the National Board for Health and Welfare (Socialstyrelsen; SS) and the Civil Contingency Agency (Myndigheten för samhällskydd och beredskap; MSB). In Denmark, and to some extent in Norway, the government should also have acted upon recommendations of the respective health authorities, which did not speak so much in favour of strict measures such as universal lockdowns or border closures. In this context, special legislative amendments were passed in all haste to put politicians more firmly in the driver's seat, and Norway went through a comparable process. In Sweden the institutional equilibrium made it more difficult to do the same, but the political situation also played a role in this respect, with a weak Red–Green coalition government led by Social Democrat Stefan Löfven that rested on a minority coalition and on a fragile agreement with some of the opposition parties.

- While many countries entered some type of state of emergency or passed special legislation that became the new normal in 2020, Sweden has no emergency provisions for peacetime (Cameron and Jonsson-Cornell, 2020). It more or less followed the standard operating procedures in case of extraordinary events and epidemics. This implies coordination among many levels, in particular with regional and local governments as well as the private contractors that assume significant responsibility for health care and elderly care services. The Swedish constitution also enshrines protection against deprivation of liberties and guarantees freedom of movement (Jonung, 2020). This said, it should be remembered that the Danish constitution does not include much more by way of emergency provisions, yet parliament unanimously adopted amendments that transferred responsibility to the government in 12 hours, making possible unprecedented restrictions of civil rights (Cedervall Lauta, 2020). Sweden also had options to amend its law or pass a new one, which was actually done months later. Besides, past experiences demonstrated that the government could overstep its prerogatives in exceptional circumstances, most notably to save lives, but that was a political decision involving exposure to liability (Jonsson-Cornell and Salminen, 2018).

- Decentralization is an essential component of a response that is expected to follow national guidelines and recommendations issued primarily by FHM but also by the main government agency under the Ministry of Health (SS). Primary care services and nursing homes are essentially organized at the municipal level, while hospitals are managed by the provinces (Landsting) with six health regions that coordinate resources. There are only a few privately run hospitals, but local governments have increasingly contracted out care services, especially for the elderly (Blomqvist and Winblad, 2020). Decentralization is also the norm for crisis management during extraordinary events. Each municipal and county council should have a specific board in charge but, as we will see, emergency plans were often missing or failed (Becker and Bynander, 2017).

- One last element that may set Sweden apart in this context is the relatively high level of trust in government agencies and in specialized expertise. In spite of mounting controversies about the national strategy and rising mortality, organizations such as FHM and their representatives enjoyed approval rates that rarely went below 60% during most of the crisis (Helsingen et al, 2020).

With this basic context in mind, it becomes easier to make some sense of the Swedish conduct throughout the pandemic. It is within this framework that the different actors involved and, more generally, the Swedish people, evaluated the new threat and responded on the basis of the recommendations provided by public agencies. In the early phase, the general impression was still that of an orderly process of crisis management led by cold-blooded decision makers, aloof from the sense of panic that seemed to predominate in many other countries at the beginning of March 2020. But it is important to recall that while northern Italy was already beset by the virus at the time, Sweden had not yet counted its first casualty. Denmark, which was hit a little before Sweden, started to react more forcefully. The government of Mette Frederiksen ordered a two-week lockdown on 11 March and closed all borders to most foreigners and tourists on 13 March. Large-scale events such as the highly popular Eurovision song contest were eventually held without an audience in Denmark, but not in Stockholm, where a similar event took place as planned with nearly 30,000 in attendance on 7 March.

The Swedish authorities have been blamed for underestimating the gravity of the threat at the time or for making dubious prognoses about the pandemic's development, but they otherwise abided by the principles and norms that govern crisis management. At first glance it seems to be in stark contrast with the idea of an 'organizational crisis' several social scientists have put forward to describe, for instance, the French approach in 2020. In this particular case, ad hoc expert committees were created in haste all around the executive branch, and the normal channels of response were partly sidelined. This centralization ran the obvious risk of concentrating all the blame, but it made possible a radically new policy of universal lockdown that was decided upon within a few days in early

March (Bergeron et al., 2020; Bandelow et al, 2021). The spread of lockdowns as a standard crisis mode across many countries was indeed striking. On the other hand, there were organizational problems more typical of the Swedish system, such as the high degree of autonomy of agencies and a disparity in interpreting and implementing national guidelines locally as well as problems of coordination in a fragmented landscape.

Before turning to the interactions between actors in the field of crisis, it is perhaps in order to recall some of the main measures and recommendations issued in Sweden in response to the new state of pandemic declared by the WHO on 11 March 2020. The day before, the level of risk in Sweden had been reassessed to 'very high', which led to a set of new regulations within a week: public gatherings of more than 500 people were forbidden (later in March, the limit was reduced to 50),[2] university, high school and adult remote education was recommended (and even remote work in the Stockholm area), the qualifying period for sick pay was suspended, in order to induce workers with symptoms to stay at home, and nonessential travel to Sweden was temporarily banned. Domestic travel remained possible but was expected to be limited, yet ski resorts remained open throughout March and only 'crowding' was to be avoided in places such as bars and restaurants. Visits to nursing homes were not formally discontinued until 31 March but could be on a local basis. In the first daily press briefings held by the trio of public agencies, the goal of protecting the frail elderly was firmly repeated, yet it was not at all clear how the responsible services and relatives should adjust, except for washing hands, keeping distances and reducing visits. The questions of tests or lack thereof was also part of the problem, since it was decided early on to focus testing on people presenting symptoms, sending an unclear message to those in close contact with vulnerable persons.

In the daily press briefing on 17 March, state epidemiologist Anders Tegnell said that this was only the tip of a gigantic iceberg and that national statistics were probably just a faint reflection of the real spread of the virus. Protecting the vulnerable was going to be "the absolutely most important thing we can do together to reduce the burden of the epidemic on the health care system and on society at large".[3] FHM issued a number of guidelines, some of which were directly transcribed into legislation. But they relied on many actors at different levels, public and private, as well as trusting the public to do the right thing. The number of controls that could be carried out was limited, and Sweden did not make extensive use of either contact tracing or police patrols of the type that issued more than two million fines in France in 2020.

It is important next to identify more precisely the main actors in charge of the response, the division of work between them and some of the assumptions, anticipations and choices they made that proved decisive.

Actors on the scene: shaping the response to COVID-19

In spite of an apparent respect for the legal framework and constraints that govern crisis management in Sweden, it is possible to argue that a few actors came to play an extraordinary role much beyond what is usually expected of them, even in exceptional circumstances. This phenomenon arose from the controversies that the Swedish case sparked in international media and politics, giving unusual visibility to certain experts and bureaucrats who normally remain in the shadows and who were suddenly pushed very hard to justify their choices. In this almost surreal context, the responsibility principle that privileges continuity in the division of labour between organizations in case of a crisis – to avoid giving far-reaching authority to specific actors (Becker and Bynander, 2017, p 8) – was put to a severe test. Indeed, the FHM team achieved unprecedented influence over the design of the response and also over crisis communication – sometimes well beyond the official channels in Sweden – although they certainly did not have enough resources or power to monitor implementation of their recommendations on all levels. In this sense, the larger nationwide response and its potential failings were the result of the fragile transmission chain, whereby local actors enjoy considerable freedom in following the guidelines. Moreover, it seems that the unusual political configuration with a weak government and a prime minister who was not so eager to take the lead, whereas several experts had strong personalities and convictions, also reinforced the traditional division of responsibilities in favour of the expert bureaucracy. The latter already played a key role in the management of the H1N1 crisis (swine flu) in 2009–2010. This time, the risk was that scientific experts would be transformed into political – and even diplomatic – actors by default (Baekkeskov and Rubin, 2014).

Crisis preparedness

Anyone who watched a single one of the Swedish daily COVID-19 media briefings could identify the traditional trio of organizations in charge of the response, although it was not easy to understand the responsibilities of each one. Because of the nature of the crisis, FHM and its duet of state epidemiologists, Anders Tegnell and (adjunct) Anders Wallensteen, obviously took the leading role. Together or alternately they have been in charge of updates on the development of the epidemic in Sweden and abroad and of announcing the evolution of recommendations and specific policies to tackle the virus. They quickly became the public face of the response, for foreign media also, even though the actual director of FHM was Johan Carlsson. By their side were the spokespersons for two other important organizations I have already mentioned: the SS, the main body responsible for health care and social care in the country, and the MSB, which is in charge of public safety in emergencies. The turnover of spokespersons at press briefings has been more frequent for the latter agencies, so that it is more difficult to identify them with one single familiar face. Both FHM and SS are direct emanations of the Ministry of Health and Social Affairs, but in line with the Swedish constitution they enjoy a high degree of autonomy in their actions. Moreover, FHM was created in 2014 as a merger of the Swedish Institute for Communicable Disease Control and the National Public Health Institute, assuming responsibilities that had belonged to SS before. It became the principal agent in charge of public health and transmissible diseases, with Dr Johan Carlson, an infectious disease specialist, as its general director since the merger. The predecessors of this institution (Svenska bakteriologiska laboratorium then Smittskyddsinstitutet) enjoyed a worldwide reputation for expertise in the fields of epidemiology and vaccines. Yet the recent administrative restructuring may have led to some of FHM's scientific competence being dispersed across universities instead (Anderberg, 2021, p 46).

Anders Tegnell, a phlegmatic physician, was born in 1956. Trained in tropical medicine, he had been appointed state epidemiologist in the new agency, but he had been around for quite some time. The story goes that, after practising for a while in Africa, Tegnell was recruited by one of the father figures of Swedish epidemiology, Johan Giesecke, at the end of the 1990s. Giesecke saw in Tegnell an unusual capacity to resist stress and pressure (Anderberg, 2021, p 21). Indeed, this may well have proven to be one of his strongest assets some 20 years down the road when COVID-19 made its breakthrough. Never before, I assume, was a Swedish bureaucrat put under so much pressure and worldwide media coverage. In any case, he worked in a milieu of specialists in a relatively small country of less than ten million, with close professional relationships in the Nordic and European regions. In 2005, the European Centre for Disease Prevention and Control (ECDC) was established in a suburb of Stockholm, with Giesecke as one of the architects. Everyone knew each other well in the small community of experts, and some were very close, to the point that Giesecke himself was asked by his former apprentice, Tegnell, if he did not want to come out of retirement and support FHM in a consulting role in March 2020. Together, their influence on the Swedish COVID-19 strategy and communication surrounding it became significant. Giesecke was indeed very vocal in both Swedish and foreign media about the choices made at the beginning of the crisis, convinced as he was that Sweden had done the right thing and that other countries imposing strict lockdowns would merely defer infections and experience trouble deciding when and how to reopen until treatments or vaccines were available.[4]

The representation of a liberal Sweden in spring 2020 may be counterpoised with the very different approach to risk in previous epidemics in this country, as Peter Baldwin rightly pointed out (Baldwin, 2021). It is not necessary to go back in time as far as cholera, but the episode of swine flu in 2009 was one of the last instances of elevated risk and one that certainly had an impact on the Swedish approach in 2020. At the time, Tegnell and FHM director Carlson already occupied comparable positions, the former being responsible for the decision to recommend mass vaccination of the Swedish population. Almost six million Swedes eventually received the Pandemrix vaccine injection, whereas other countries such as Denmark adopted a more targeted strategy. France also preventively secured a high number of doses but stopped short, vaccinating no more than 7% of the population. This episode most likely left an imprint on later strategies for preparedness in countries that may have overestimated the risk, and with potentially serious side-effects of the vaccine. Besides, the rise of other global threats such as terrorism also led to a certain degree of priority shifts and to an organizational drift that affected some of the strategic reserves of material maintained to confront a pandemic (Bergeron et al, 2020, p 20).

In any case, pandemic preparedness was certainly suboptimal in Sweden, as in most countries, and even before 2009. In 2008, a report of the National Audit Office (Riksrevision) had reviewed plans in three counties – including Stockholm – as well as in 69 communes. It found that only a handful had planned for this type of exceptional crisis. Even Karolinska Hospital, one of the largest in Europe, was found to lack a specific road map. Local governments and institutions enjoyed a high degree of freedom to organize, but responsibilities and resources were spread widely and unequally, with an overall deficit of national coordination. The National Audit Office considered 'the shortcomings observed during the audit to be so numerous and, in some cases, so serious that there may not be time to put them right before the [swine flu] pandemic reaches Sweden'.[5] Setting up a proper public health agency through the merger of different services in 2014 formed part of the response to some of these coordination failings, but the reform did not entail local governments and care services significantly stepping up their efforts to ensure better preparedness.

In addition, the capacity for civil response to a crisis that was entrusted to MSB was arguably more limited than before, when Sweden had a so-called doctrine of 'total defence' (Engberg, 2004). Gradually dismantled in the wake of the Cold War, it was slowly revamped after the annexation of Crimea by Russia in 2014, and in 2018, in parallel with the reinstatement of national conscription, MSB had sent a brochure to Swedish citizens to guide them in case of war or severe crisis.[6]

Sweden ranked seventh in the 2019 Global Health Security Index that measures health security and capabilities, with a low score for emergency preparedness and response planning or operations. However, the two countries that ranked first and second in the world were the US and the UK, which, as it happened, were equally overwhelmed by the pandemic. Finland, ranking last of the top ten, was better prepared in terms of supplies of material, such as masks, having learned the hard lesson of being cornered in the Baltic Sea on the front lines of the Cold War for decades. Sweden had relaxed controls on its stocks after 1989 and in the process of European integration. In 2009, the state pharmaceutical service was privatized and supply became even more dependent on market mechanisms functioning well (Andersson and Pryser Libell, 2020). Yet Sweden's capacity did not seem to be the only reason for its policy toward testing or mask wearing in the initial phase of the pandemic, even though masks and other resources were clearly lacking for exposed professionals and vulnerable persons. It was also the result of a conviction at FHM that mass testing was less effective once circulation of the virus was high, that its cost was significant and that masks were improperly used by the general public, giving a false sense of security.[7] Indeed, a couple of months passed before Sweden reached a testing level on a par with the actual capacity of the country. Though the Ministry of Health set a goal of stepping up testing significantly at the end of March 2020, the number of tests carried out remained at a fraction of the potential up until the summer, reflecting difficulties in the implementation chain at the regional level. While Sweden is usually in line with recommendations of the WHO, it clearly departed from the early injunction of its general director to test as much as possible. In this area, the government, FHM and local government conveniently blamed each other for the delay.

Herd immunity

One of the main questions that was raised with respect to the COVID-19 crisis was to what extent and why the Swedish official strategy of mitigation actually relied on the hope to achieve some form of herd immunity in the spring of 2020. Journalist Johannes Anderberg recently published book in Swedish on this topic, provocatively entitled *The Herd* (Anderberg, 2021), draws on interviews and on the correspondence among some of the key actors in the crisis, attempting to put together the scattered pieces that eventually composed the Swedish strategy. This work details the personal ties and contacts in a tightly knit community of scientific experts and civil servants in Sweden and beyond, and it casts light on the circumstances and assumptions that specifically informed the Swedish approach. More academic contributions to this discussion of the Swedish idiosyncrasy have started to appear and will be brought into the discussion.

One of the turning points in the process was the impact and interpretation of the report of the Imperial College COVID-19 Response Team, authored by British epidemiologist Neil Ferguson and colleagues. Formally published on 16 March 2020, it began to circulate a few days earlier and played an important role in the policy shifts in countries such as the UK and France. The summary of the report started with this chilling sentence: 'The global impact of COVID-19 has been profound, and the public health threat it represents is the most serious seen in a respiratory virus since the 1918 H1N1 influenza pandemic.' While the report acknowledged that the current context was very different from that of 1918, it nonetheless predicted potentially very high numbers of casualties, nearing half a million in the UK, if strict policies to suppress the virus were not implemented swiftly (Ferguson et al, 2020).

At that time, the British options seemed to matter a lot to Sweden. Although Boris Johnson and his government could not be regarded as the best example of caution and preparation in the pandemic – to say the least – they apparently lent precious support to the emerging strategy of mitigation in Sweden. It is established that Swedish experts at FHM and around it, some of whom knew Ferguson well and had collaborated with him, considered that the report exhibited a number of flaws that made its forecast dubious. It assumed, among other things, that hospital capacity was inflexible – especially for intensive care – and that a majority of people would not sufficiently adjust their conduct or follow the rules of self-isolation in case of symptoms unless forced to do so (Anderberg, 2021, p 126). At the foundation of the report lay estimates of virus transmission and mortality that were derived mostly from Chinese data and that lent themselves to discussion. The history of pandemic alerts is also riddled with dreadful predictions that thankfully proved to be mistaken many times. Therefore, it was not difficult to cast doubt on the report even though its influence was considerable on decisions to lock down.

However, the decisive arguments – if any – in the Swedish context appeared to be that the consequences of the 'suppression strategy' (i.e., strict lockdown) were not only unpredictable but potentially serious in the long run and that it would be particularly difficult to impose stay-at-home orders on legal and constitutional grounds (Jonsson-Cornell and Salminen, 2018; Jonung, 2020). Hence the official reasoning by mid-March 2020 had two goals: to slow down the spread of the virus and to protect the most vulnerable. If the degree of success in meeting the first goal is open to discussion, the second one clearly met with failure in light of the skyrocketing mortality in nursing homes, especially in the capital region.

General population lockdown has not been the most common policy option in the modern arsenal against pandemics and is regarded as a thing of the past. The swiftness with which it was adopted in a number of countries as far away as India was therefore surprising, and Swedish authorities could thus claim that they were actually following a well-established strategy of mitigation, in coherence with the pandemic preparation plan of 2019 that clearly identified both the goals and the responsible actors: 'Preparation plans for pandemic influenza shall reduce adverse consequences and strive to limit the spread of infection. Folkhälsomyndigheten (FHM) oversees pandemic preparedness at the national level and gives support to planning at the regional and local levels.'[8]

As I mentioned at the start of this section, much of the controversy has revolved around the extent to which FHM and the Swedish government consciously supported a search for some kind of 'herd immunity' under the official label of mitigation. This concept has become the epicentre of the Swedish story, with the strangely negative connotation associated with the notion of 'herd' that symbolically equates human societies with animal groupings. Yet formally the concept refers solely to the level of immunity, achieved by antibodies and/or through vaccines, that indirectly protects people who are not yet immune. At the end of the day, this is the goal that every nation should hope for, one that is not at all certain to be achieved on a global scale even with the help of vaccines. In an open world and with highly unequal rates of transmission and vaccination, experts now believe that it is fairly unlikely in the near future (Aschwanden, 2021; Mandavili, 2021). However, the level of uncertainty about the virus and the development of treatments or vaccines was obviously much higher in spring 2020, meaning decision makers had to rely on hypotheses not only about infection patterns but also about the behaviour and discipline of citizens, which in turn were influenced by the nature of public recommendations and policies (Capano et al, 2020).

In his book about the first wave, Peter Baldwin argues that there is a contradiction between a search for natural herd immunity and recommendations to work from home whenever possible, limit mobility to the essential and self-quarantine in case of any symptom, which summed up the main Swedish recommendations in the spring (Baldwin, 2021, p 145). Experts in Stockholm may have anticipated rising immunity thanks to the continuous circulation of the virus, but the FHM team publicly denied that it was more than a by-product. They nonetheless expressed contradictory opinions, especially in their correspondence (Anderberg, 2021, p 94; Eriksson et al, 2020). It was probably not realistic to believe that immunity would reach levels in the vicinity of 50% or more within a couple of months while Swedes voluntarily limited their interactions almost in the proportion of Denmark, where stricter measures had been passed. All the more since FHM considered that the virus was primarily not airborne. FHM expected rates of about 20% in May only in Stockholm, but the first antibody studies reported disappointingly low rates of immunity in the capital, close to 8% (Henley, 2020b). These results should have sent a warning sign to the Swedish authorities, but they came at a time when the epidemic was already on the way down, before summer 2020, so that it did not modify the official discourse and policy.

In public debate, the opposition of two simplistic 'strategies', namely lockdown vs. (natural) herd immunity, has been misleading. It conveyed a wrong image that some countries were putting up a strong fight to suppress the virus whereas others – such as Sweden – were just letting it run loose and waiting for some degree of natural immunity. In truth, only a few countries managed to keep the virus at bay in the first wave through strict quarantines and sophisticated contact tracing policies. Most of the others relied on an array of measures that were effective only in so far as institutions and people accepted and followed them and in so far as health care infrastructures could withstand the shock. In this context, Sweden distinguished itself by resorting to a form of mitigation policy based on recommendations that looked all the more liberal because a majority of countries were implementing legally binding stay-at-home orders on a grand scale.

In Chapter Three, I will return to the controversy surrounding herd immunity, but through the lens of the extensive international media coverage and of the heated debate it stirred inside and outside Sweden.

Political abdication?

With epidemiologists turning into political actors, one might well wonder what Swedish politicians did, at least during this first wave. In comparison to most other countries, the relative invisibility of political leadership in Sweden was a rather striking phenomenon – seen from outside – and raises important comparative questions. One interpretation is that the political elite stuck to the rulebook and let the expert bureaucracy take charge, as it should according to the Swedish division of responsibilities (Baekkeskov and Rubin, 2014). Agencies such as FHM would issue recommendations, for example, to shut down air transport between Sweden and Iran at the beginning of March, and the responsible ministry services or local government would respond accordingly. Not only does the constitution limit the possibilities of direct ministerial orders to a given public administration, but the doctrine in crisis situations also prescribes an orderly response in line with the prerogatives of each level of the Swedish institutions (Becker and Bynander, 2017). The key factor that might hold such a pyramid together was said to be a high level of social and political trust. Indeed, this was by and large the message captured in the parliamentary questions to the prime minister on 17 March 2020. The first speech by Ulf Kristersson, leader of the Conservative Party, stressed that a spirit of solidarity and trust in the government was essential and that "it is a Swedish tradition in times of crisis that we cooperate to solve problems, and we leave political quarrels to the side".[9] Later in this debate, Prime Minister Lövfen very clearly expressed that "all the decisions that the government makes ... we want them to be made according to the expert authorities". These words set the stage for what would be the trademark of political action for the greater part of 2020, and maybe even after. This debate also incorporated most of the typical properties of the Swedish parliamentary practice: it was apparently orderly and respectful, collaborative and responsible.

However, in this exceptional context, it was easy to forget that Swedish politics had been in a crisis of its own for some time, at least since Stefan Löfven himself first took office in 2014. With the rise of a national populist party in the 2000s, the Sweden Democrats (SverigeDemokraterna; SD), the share of other political forces has shrunk. It has become increasingly difficult to form a government on the premise that SD should be permanently excluded from power at the national level. They have made significant inroads into local politics and succeeded in cornering the mainstream parties into awkward agreements between Left and Right in Parliament. The current minority government headed by the Social Democrats and in coalition with the Green Party is thus in a rather weak position. Prime Minister Stefan Löfven was himself not the kind of personality who fancies the political limelight. He was surprisingly the first Social Democratic prime minister in Swedish history with a background as a worker and trade union leader and no prior political mandate. In addition, he became leader of the party by default. He had a tendency to shun the media and was keen to leave the gist of crisis management and communication to the experts at FHM (Anderberg, 2021, p 72). His relationship to unions and more broadly to industrial interests might also help explain why he could easily support the goal of keeping most sectors of the economy running. Yet the evolution of Swedish social democracy and the dependence of his government on a fragile parliamentary balance with the Centre-Right parties could also make his cabinet more receptive to business interests. The minister of health and social affairs, 47-year-old Lena Hallengren, was a pure product of the Social Democratic meritocracy. She had limited responsibilities related to health care before her appointment in autumn 2019 to replace a minister who had resigned, though she held the portfolio for children and the elderly for a few months. She was thus new to the field in many ways when the pandemic struck and perhaps did not have either the experience or the legitimacy to play a more decisive role.

These more contingent elements have to be factored in to make sense of the Swedish response. It certainly does not imply that the political elites were utterly passive. Compared to many other countries – even the Nordic ones – they were not as visible, but it has to be seen in a Swedish context. Stefan Löfven delivered a short address to the nation on 22 March 2020. It was the first instance since the assassination of Foreign Minister Anna Lindh in 2002 of such a speech by a prime minister. On this occasion, he stated: "I, as prime minister, and the government I lead, will take every decision that is necessary to protect the lives, health and jobs of as many people as we possibly can."[10] A crisis organization at the cabinet level did exist, a so-called Group for Strategic Coordination housed in Mikael Damberg's Ministry of the Interior that first met at the end of January. State Secretary Elisabeth Backteman, who had the responsibility for this group, did not have any specific background or expertise in health-related fields and almost none of the participants would ever make public appearances during the crisis. Backteman was referred to in the media as an unknown bureaucrat bearing a heavy responsibility (Kullberg, 2020). She had a small staff at her disposal and also led a Crisis Council that had been created as a result of the failure to handle the human consequences of the 2004 tsunami in Southeast Asia, when many Swedes lost their lives or had to be repatriated. The report of the special commission of inquiry on this particular event had already underlined the weaknesses of political coordination in times of crisis.[11]

Here we start to see the larger picture of the infrastructure dealing with the crisis – but only at the national level. It was an assemblage of organizations that operated within a typical Swedish institutional framework but that had also been impacted in one way or another by previous and recent experiences of crisis management, ranging from a tsunami to the swine flu threat. Sweden has a tradition of setting up commissions to investigate this type of event, and some of them manage to have a bearing on the actual organization and preparedness. As Becker and Bynander stress:

> The government has over the last ten years increased its ability to exercise this responsibility, by creating functions in the ministries and the government offices as a whole to deal with strategic and normative issues at the national level. There are, however, many vertical gaps in responsibility that can lead to time lags and confusion as to responsibilities during large scale crisis that demands a wide coordination effort at the national level. (Becker and Bynander, 2017, p 14)

Reflecting on the recent work by Bergeron and his colleagues regarding the case of France, we do not see a comparable level of 'organizational saturation' or complexity that becomes a problem in times of crisis (Bergeron et al, 2020), and very few new entities were devised on this occasion except for the purpose of public inquiry. Yet Sweden nevertheless faced important coordination problem in a regime that is not based on a highly hierarchical power pyramid but rather on a constellation of territories and a kind of 'soft governance'. It is obviously an immense task to respond to a new challenge of such magnitude, but the organizing principles of crisis management that do not shift responsibilities to one central command, do not create new layers or kludges and rely on the 'normal' division of labour stand in contrast with the experience of many other countries. Swedish authorities had undoubtedly taken stock from severe warnings in the last 15 years and tried to improve coordination between units and levels. There was even some work underway with a government commission reviewing preparedness in the health sector and considering a pandemic scenario as one of the possibilities.[12] However, the degree of decentralization and fragmentation as well as the systemic overload in this specific field made an ageing society particularly vulnerable to a shock of this brutality and magnitude.

As the virus took its toll in the spring, decimating elderly people and especially those in nursing homes in Sweden, and as opposition to the official line started to mount, the government resorted to soliciting extraordinary powers in April that could be granted by Parliament only on a temporary basis. The rationale was to be able to quickly implement selective shutdown of public or private services or venues if it was deemed necessary. The Communicable Disease Act allowed for some forms of interventions to protect the population, but it was then considered preferable to amend it and add new dispositions tailored to the pandemic. On 18 April 2020, Parliament voted on a list of six specific types of measures to be used for a duration of less than three months.[13] There was absolutely no blank cheque to the government that had hoped for more substantial powers. New regulations were not to infringe on the fundamental rights protected by the constitution and any substantial limit on the freedom of movement, such as a curfew, would have required an entirely new law. Furthermore, the government did not enjoy the ability to act alone and had to submit any new proposal to Parliament for speedy review (Jonasson and Larue, 2020, pp 4–5). In the end, the Swedish government did not ever use its newly acquired powers.

As we can see, the checks and balances in Sweden constrained political action, arguably to a much greater extent than in many other countries where emergency powers could be granted, special legislation passed and new organizations created more easily. However, the Danish constitution does not explicitly refer to a state of emergency either and thus does not depart so fundamentally from the Swedish case, even though the autonomy of public agencies is not as entrenched. Yet the government of Mette Frederiksen also enjoyed a stronger position than its neighbour and stepped in early in March to have Parliament change the Epidemic Act in order to implement a series of strict but temporary restrictions and to transfer certain responsibilities to the state level. As noted earlier, the Danish Public Health Agency was not initially in full agreement with such strict measures, but the government managed to bypass it. Finland is another example of strong administrative autonomy – in line with the Swedish model – that did not prevent the executive from taking the lead in the crisis (Jonsson-Cornell and Salminen, 2018; Bentzen et al, 2020). In comparison, the Swedish FHM was certainly eager to assert its prerogatives and made that very clear to Parliament when the possibility of granting more power to the government in spring 2020 was contemplated (Andersson and Aylott, 2020).

A combination of elements thus factored into the production of the response observed in Sweden: beyond the legal framework and traditional division of responsibilities which assigned a key role to agencies and local government, the weakness of the minority cabinet and the profiles of certain political leaders and their staff – particularly the prime minister and minister of health – made the government more likely to rely on seasoned experts in this exceptional crisis. Among them were strong personalities with prior experience of epidemic risks and an assessment of the situation that made them beware of overreaction. However, what was presented as respect for the constitution, for civil rights and liberties and for scientific expertise may equally well come to be regarded as fragile political responsibility and leadership, lack of capacity to react to an emergency or even as delegation of democratic power to bureaucratic experts. The government initiative to promote more testing in the spring of 2020 is a good example of the multiple constraints that paved the way of political ambitions: tests and lab capacity had to be available, FHM was not fully convinced that it was a priority once the epidemic was widespread, and local authorities took time to comply with the objective and deliver. The high level of pluralism and delegation in this parliamentary democracy has led to a dilution of responsibilities along with the intriguing paradox of the emergence of one highly visible actor, namely state epidemiologist Anders Tegnell.

THREE

Comparing Nations in a World Crisis

One of the many paradoxes of the coronavirus pandemic crisis was to produce an historic retrenchment of states within national borders: governments closed off entries and exits while opening up a wave of comparisons of national strategies, policies and performance in the battle against this virus. Never before had there been so much sudden interest in comparing expert recommendations, political responses and the health statistics compiled on a daily basis. In a matter of weeks, by March 2020, our daily lives became saturated with infection and death rates and measures of hospitalizations and intensive care beds. To be sure, not all countries were on a level playing field in terms of health care infrastructure or even statistical capacity to measure the real impact of the COVID-19. The degree of exposure to the virus also varied tremendously over space and time, but it did not seem to matter much to the mediasphere, social networks or other databases that fed us on a continuous and gigantic flow of information and statistics throughout 2020. Comparisons were also meant as a form of benchmarking between countries, sometimes with heavily moral evaluations. Because the advanced Western welfare states were hit early on and quite severely, they remained more evidently in the spotlight, but comparisons were commonly made with countries such as Taiwan, Israel, South Africa or Peru in various regions of the world. As a consequence, the pandemic expanded our horizons on the one hand while narrowing them drastically on the other because of border closings and local quarantines or lockdowns.

Another striking characteristic of this crisis was the blending of scientific, political and popular judgements about the pandemic and the various national responses it triggered. In its magnitude, it became the first global event during the era of digital media and social networks to so intensely affect people's daily lives in so many countries at once. Previous pandemic flu episodes of a similar nature during the 1950s and 1960s mostly went under the radar, in spite of estimated mortality that was significant. In 2020, the situation was very different: digital media and networks became a springboard for opinions of all kinds blended together. The degree of novelty and uncertainty associated with the virus and its consequences led to a relative devaluation of scientific and expert discourse as compared to political and popular opinion, accompanied by the rapid spread of various rumours and conspiracy theories. This climate of post-truth found significant support in the very leadership of the biggest democratic countries, such as the US under Donald Trump, Brazil under Jair Bolsonaro and India under Narendra Modi, but also in more authoritarian regimes. At the same time, never before had lay people had such easy access to statistical data and also to scientific and medical information, laying bare the controversies and conflicts of interests inherent in the construction of modern science and pharmaceutical interests. In this respect, the controversy surrounding the effectiveness of a treatment based on the combination of well-known and inexpensive hydroxychloroquine and azithromycin, launched by French infectious disease specialist Didier Raoult in spring 2020, was one of the best illustrations of the changing status of scientific debate and evidence (Berlivet and Löwy, 2020).

Sweden occupies a special and very ambivalent position in this picture. As I have argued, the foreign representations of the Swedish model are usually overwhelmingly positive and associated with progress although they incorporate a degree of ambivalence. In its regular reports on Swedish image in international media, the Swedish Institute aptly and simply sums it up: 'Sweden is conceived of as a democratic, peaceful and secure country governed in a skillfull and honest fashion. Sweden is also regarded as a country where the freedoms and rights of citizens are respected, and where equality is important' (Svenska Institutet, 2020, p. 3). Over time, Swedes have shrewdly capitalized on this image. Sweden's reputation also rested on the capacity of a small country to stand its ground in the midst of great power rivalries, drawing from a practice of nonalignment and a commitment to peace-building (Brommesson, 2018). At the same time, the kind of soft socialism practised in Sweden always had detractors, and, as the country moved toward more neoliberal reforms of its welfare system, criticism started to come from the Left as well. Hence the status of the Swedish model brand has become more blurred recently, with symbolic and ideological battles over its positive or negative values. In this sense, what Paul Rapacioli described as a 'good Sweden–bad Sweden' duality is becoming more prominent in social media (Rapacioli, 2018b).

The pandemic doubtless gave a radically new dimension to this duality, bending opinions much more clearly toward the negative side, to the opposite of progress, welfare and social care that constitute the backbone of the classical Swedish model, but much less so for the democratic rights and liberties that were preserved. Because of the great uncertainty that prevailed in 2020, the Swedish deviation became a primary site of controversy. There was arguably no other place in the world that attracted so much attention and passion for a time, though the US under Trump probably came close. What Sweden embodied in the public eye was a fundamental conflict between individual freedom and collective security that raised two important questions. The first was not so much whether Swedes could escape all restrictions on their basic freedoms but whether these restrictions were to be mandated by the state or made dependent on individual will; the second was whether the welfare and health system was strong enough to absorb the pandemic shock and to guarantee good access to care and compensation for all.

In the COVID-19 crisis, Sweden thus played the role of the outlier to which other national policies could be compared: Were they politically legitimate, efficient at limiting infection as well as mortality, and eventually morally defensible? Trying to answer these difficult questions implied drawing selectively from different aspects of what is usually perceived as the Swedish model in order to reconstruct a narrative that was contradictory or coherent with it. The relatively high flexibility of this model framework and its recent evolutions made it possible to do this and to reconsider Sweden as a much more ambivalent political and welfare example. The pandemic response also had a strong impact on domestic debates in a country where the expression of dissent is perhaps more constrained than in other democracies, especially in times of crisis. On both fronts, nationally and internationally, Swedish public authorities were unusually active in justifying their actions and limiting collateral damage to their reputations. Once again, state epidemiologist Anders Tegnell, assisted by his staff, was one of the main agents in charge of communication, even if members of the government also played a role. Beyond the daily briefings in which Tegnell patiently answered questions from Swedish and foreign journalists, he gave countless interviews and turned into the type of controversial pop icon that Swedish environmental activist Greta Thunberg had become in recent years. In September 2020, The British *Sun* tabloid newspaper was even reporting on his status of 'national hero' (Harvey, 2020). This conversion of an obscure bureaucrat and medical expert to a status of near stardom, with a Facebook fan-page and t-shirts bearing his likeness – but equally strong expressions of hate – was an unexpected and striking phenomenon. It conveyed the real extent and strength of national sentiments lurking behind the health care strategies.

The main goal of this chapter is to show why and how Sweden played such a prominent role in the comparison of and controversies around pandemic response strategies across the world. During the crisis, there was a specific framing of the controversies about Sweden that built on the role and image that this country has carved out for itself in international politics. I document the evolution of references to the Swedish case, how they were used and how they were sometimes twisted to legitimize or criticize not just the Swedish line but also other national strategies in return.

The sheer novelty of 2020 was that negative judgments progressively outnumbered positive ones, with Sweden becoming something of an anti-model – even a 'pariah state' not to be emulated, though there were die-hard supporters as well (Erdbrink, 2020). As a consequence, Swedish public officials and diplomats had to wage a real war of communication to justify their choices, but they regularly went further by claiming that their approach would prove more pragmatic and more legitimate in the long run. This type of attitude and the waves of criticism that ensued from abroad fuelled a strange form of 'public health nationalism' in Sweden, with Anders Tegnell and Johan Giesecke as the main spokespersons facing sometimes violent controversies at home. The justifications put forward by public officials and supporters often resorted to some basic elements and values of the model discourse, but they came under mounting pressure both from within and outside the country. Finally, the Swedish deviation within the Nordic region also paved the way for regional tensions that will be reviewed in more detail further on.

The analysis builds on an abundance of domestic and foreign media sources on the Swedish strategy from spring to summer 2020. The fragmented and changing representation of Sweden appears to be dependent on the origin and type of publication but also on sequences of opinion-building that led to increased polarization within and outside Sweden in spring 2020. This crisis also had a tremendous effect on both the form and content of communication and on the status of some actors, with state epidemiologist Anders Tegnell becoming the public face of Sweden.

The battle for public opinion

No quantitative analysis is needed to show that the Swedish anomaly ranked high in international media coverage of COVID-19 in 2020. Suffice it to say that the Swedish Institute, which extensively surveys foreign opinion and images of Sweden, had never in modern times seen such high interest (Eriksson, 2020c; Laurén, 2020). Countries that imposed strict quarantines and boasted good results, like Taiwan, South Korea or New Zealand, also garnered world interest. Conversely, the 'ostrich' league, including Brazil, the US (then, later, some of the US states) or even the UK for a short time, also made the headlines. But several things clearly made Sweden stand out. The first was its status as a social democratic welfare state and its international reputation not only as an advanced welfare regime but also as a 'moral superpower' that often promoted a different stance in international politics (Ingebritsen, 2006). The second was the decision against strict lockdown of the population and against a general mask mandate later in spring 2020 when a majority of European countries were privileging strategies of containment. I would add at least a third reason, which lies in the specific style of crisis communication adopted by Swedish decision makers and particularly official experts: the awkward combination of placidity and some degree of resignation in the face of rising mortality with something that at times came to be seen as superiority or arrogance and was deeply troubling.

The uses of Swedish exceptionalism

One predominant term used throughout the crisis was 'exceptional', vocabulary that echoed well the typical semantic of the Swedish model as almost unique in the democratic world (Hilson, 2008). This stems not only from its history of universal welfare provision and redistribution but also from the special role social democracy has played and from a number of political and institutional arrangements fostering public transparency and consensus-building. In spite of profound changes of the system and possibly of the values that underpin it, this mental map of Sweden is still resilient, especially in foreign representations but also at home. I personally used this vocabulary of 'exception' in an op-ed published online by the French newspaper *Libération* in early April 2020, although the website too glibly summed up my viewpoint, writing that Sweden had chosen a 'strategy of collective immunity'[1] (Aucante, 2020b). At the time, many journalists were finding what they were searching for, using keywords and labels that spread quickly and were reproduced widely. But scientists of all disciplines were also recruited in the mediasphere, multiplying and blurring the layers of meaning between expertise and opinion. There was a good deal of simplification and misunderstanding in the representation of the initial strategy that Sweden adopted and that was sometimes described as playing 'Russian roulette' by letting life go on as usual (Henley, 2020a). As Rachel Irwin argued, social life may have been less impacted than elsewhere, but it was far from normal. Many adjustments were made voluntarily by individuals and organizations. For instance, it was not the government that closed ski resorts but the operating companies, at the end of March 2020. More generally, Swedes restrained their movements and social interactions to a great extent (Irwin, 2020).

International coverage of Sweden in the initial stage of the pandemic was clearly mixed. News media had different levels of access and knowledge of the country. Some of them could rely on experienced Swedish correspondents providing nuanced reporting, such as *Le Monde*'s Anne-Françoise Hivert (France), Christian Stichler for German TV and *Die Zeit* or Richard Orange for *The Guardian*. They also testified to the increasing climate of hostility on social networks that they faced when they commented on the Swedish handling of the crisis and questioned it.[2] In addition, there were signs of rapid politicization of some national strategies against the coronavirus with the use of the Swedish example as a resource to support or discredit anti-lockdown policies. This was evident in the

UK, where newspapers such as the conservative *Daily Telegraph* regularly referred to Sweden to show that alternatives to the British strategy of lockdown might still be possible (Fenwick Elliott, 2020). *OpenDemocracy* journalist Peter Geoghegan argued that British libertarian elites that used to despise Swedish social democracy were now praising its approach in the crisis and its defence of individual freedom (Geoghegan, 2021). Ironically, even Neil Ferguson, the epidemiologist behind the famous Imperial College report that pushed Boris Johnson to change tack so fast in March 2020, was eventually caught confessing that the Swedes went 'a long way to the same effect' (Wooler, 2020). Other media such as *The Sun* published articles about Sweden nearly every week throughout 2020, and most of them were meant to find some support for British lockdown policies.

The Germans, usually quite positive toward Sweden, appeared to be more suspicious from the beginning. The country enjoyed one of the highest OECD hospital capacities, and German TV correspondent Christian Stichler repeatedly put Anders Tegnell under pressure in the daily press conferences, demanding to know what science was behind the Swedish decision to keep schools open and have so little contact tracing. FHM had for some time purported that asymptomatic cases were not the main problem, whereas Germany had started from an opposite viewpoint (Lund, 2020b; Stichler, 2020). One of the hypotheses voiced in Germany at the time was that Sweden did not have a collective memory of war and national catastrophe, and that people were not ready to make sacrifices for the greater good. Assumptions of this kind, or the mobilization of cultural stereotypes such as a German preference for hierarchy and strict instructions, became more frequent throughout the spring (Lund, 2020a; Lund, 2020c).

Tropes and sequences in opinion-building

There was a relatively consensual evolution in the foreign media with respect to Sweden in spring 2020. An extensive search of online newspapers in English, French, German, Italian and Spanish returned rather similar trends. After an initial phase of bewilderment when Sweden remained almost the only European country to shun lockdown, journalists and commentators tried to find more or less rational explanations for this apparent deviation. On 18 March, Anne-Françoise Hivert of *Le Monde* (France) wrote about 'a kingdom of irreducible Vikings to the north of a Europe that locks itself in' (Hivert, 2020a, my translation). The reference to the Vikings is a common one and is much more positive here than what history might suggest. For example, it was often used to describe the success of Icelandic financial tycoons in the period before the 2008 crash. There was an interest mixed with concern for a trajectory that was apparently based on respect of civil liberties and that could still prove to be a viable alternative to the historically severe restrictions seen in the rest of the world. As one of the main daily newspapers in hard–hit Peru stated on 28 March: 'The Swedes have followed a more liberal line than their Danish and Norwegian neighbours. But for the moment, it is not yet clear which model is the most effective.'[3] By 'effective', the journalist referred not only to health care but also to the adverse socioeconomic consequences that every country's leaders should have in the back of their minds.

However, many foreign news sources soon moved in the direction of increasing criticism of a policy that was considered far too relaxed, even irresponsible, and the opinions about Sweden became more polarized. In these reports, one could find a strange mixture of envy (Why on earth are Swedes allowed to go to the pub or gym...?) and moral judgement stemming from a mortality rate that grew more rapidly than in the other Nordic countries. On 22 March, the German *Süddeutsche Zeitung* titled an article 'the next Ischgl' in reference to the Austrian ski resort responsible for early clusters and infections of Scandinavian travellers, but also to the fact that it was still possible to go skiing in Sweden at the time. Indeed, the very idea that tourists could still flock to ski resorts in remote mountain regions with limited hospital capacities was considered evidence that Swedes were not behaving responsibly (Strittmatter, 2020). Case numbers and mortality rates – much more than measures of hospital and ICU saturation – were systematically put forward to demonstrate that the country was going to hit the wall. In other words, there must be an obvious price to pay for keeping society open and preserving some degree of freedom.[4] On 26 March, *La Repubblica* (Italy) compared the Swedish approach to what the UK and US did earlier on and considered that 'the world situation suggests an absurd and very dangerous mistake on the part of the country of the Nordic model' (Tarquini, 2020, my translation).

Apart from ski resorts, Stockholm was the epicentre of the epidemic and often seemed to be taken for the whole of Sweden. In fact, very seldom did reports document the situation in other regions. Other large cities that were apparently relatively spared during the first wave were rarely mentioned (Orange, 2020b). Some commentators, however, recalled that Swedish demography and social customs made it easier to respect distancing, that most elderly people did not live with their families in contrast to south European countries, or that Swedish cities had among the highest share of one-person dwellings (Castro, 2020). On the other hand, the situation of less well-off urban areas where communities of foreign origins resided with perhaps poorer connections to the Swedish official channels of communication and comparatively more health risk factors was also signalled. Sweden had welcomed a high number of new migrants since 2015, and the epidemic stressed both the multicultural aspect of the welfare state and the risk of ghettoization in some deprived neighbourhoods of Stockholm where overpopulated dwellings could lead to more spread (Hivert, 2020b).

From April to June, pressure mounted due to rising mortality – especially in elder care residences – and most of the international discussion started to revolve around the buzzword of 'herd immunity'. It was assumed that the authorities had let the virus spread, keeping schools and public venues open, to achieve some sort of natural immunity. The conjunction of increasing domestic criticism by some groups of scientific and medical experts who wrote open letters in the media and very divergent mortality rates among the Nordic countries led to a near consensus that the Swedish strategy had failed (Irwin, 2020). On 9 April 2020, Prime Minister Löfven gave an interview to the newspaper *Svenska Dagbladet* in which he admitted to failings in the protection of the frail elderly but also said that Sweden did not stick out so markedly from the rest of Europe in terms of mortality and each country should be allowed to follow the strategy of its choice in uncertain times (Eriksson, 2020b). Yet the lack of early and clear recommendations to the local providers of elder care services on how to protect their patients and the disparities in implementing medical and safety measures or providing protective material on the ground most likely helped spread the virus through the staff even after family visits were regulated on 1 April. Therefore, the constant underestimation of asymptomatic cases in a society where schools and other venues remained open was pointed out as a key problem by critics of the Swedish line (Orange, 2020a).

However, with no clear perspective on treatment or vaccines, this idea that societies would acquire natural immunity was still seductive in spite of its controversial nature. *New York Times* columnist Thomas L. Friedman wrote a sympathetic op-ed in late April 2020 that asked whether Sweden was not showing the hard way to go when lockdowns were exhausted:

> I believe one of the most important questions we need to answer, as these lockdowns end, is this: Are we going to adapt to the coronavirus – by design – the way Sweden is attempting to do – or are we going to go the same direction as Sweden – by messy default – or are we just going to say 'the hell with lockdowns' and go 50 different ways? (Friedman, 2020)

Friedman referred to a *New York Times* article by US physician David L. Katz that spurred the debate on the broader longer-term costs and benefits of universal lockdowns as opposed to more targeted policies focussing on risk groups and adjusting as scientific knowledge progressed (Katz, 2020). Beyond the controversial notion of herd immunity, Sweden represented a rare example of a country that seemed to put forward this broader cost–benefit analysis and, as such, it remained the darling of a surprising variety of thought groups that do not usually hold Nordic social democracy in high esteem.

The Nordic family divided

Early statements from Nordic neighbours on the Swedish response were nuanced and cautious. The people in charge in the respective public health agencies and scientific communities knew each other well and were in close contact. There was, for instance, a good deal of agreement between the Swedish agency and its Danish counterpart on border closing and to a certain extent even lockdown. Danish chief epidemiologist Søren Brodstrøm considered that the Danish government's decision to close borders as early as 13 March 2020 was a 'political' one and, as such, was not following expert advice. His Swedish colleague Anders Tegnell then commented that this decision made no sense with respect to the history of epidemic responses (Batchelor, 2020; Forsberg, 2020). There also seemed to be some agreement with Norwegian public health experts on keeping schools open. Border closing between the three Scandinavian countries was obviously a sensitive issue in a region where free movement had been the rule since the mid-1950s, resulting in significant minorities from the neighbour states and much cross-border daily commuting. To a large extent, the rules on quarantine did not apply to all those workers because they were often essential to well-functioning infrastructure. However, the policy differentials among the Nordics became a problem, and moral judgements were not far off, although there was also a tendency to refrain from officially criticizing neighbours too strongly. When Norwegians were symbolically forbidden to visit their much-loved country retreats until April 2020, those who owned properties across the Swedish border were allowed to go for one day at a time, but they later sued the state over the strict quarantine rule that applied when they returned from longer stays in Sweden. The cottage owners at first won the case in district court, but the state appealed and had the last word.

Yet the major problem was the rapidly increasing discrepancy between the Swedish COVID-19-associated mortality rates and those of other Nordic nations, the former being up to 15-fold higher during 2020, even though all-cause excess mortality may be lower than immediately perceived in Sweden (Juul et al, 2020). But the daily statistical focus on death rates accentuated the differences between countries that are otherwise relatively comparable in terms of demography, health and sociocultural profiles. Not only were the neighbours afraid of potential spread of infection from across the border, they were also shocked by the skyrocketing mortality in Sweden. The comparison with Sweden could be used to show that the other Nordics had made the right choice, and it cemented a form of national consensus – even a sense of superiority that is usually a Swedish prerogative – particularly in Norway (Moe, 2021b). Finland appeared as the other best-in-league, with a long tradition of preparedness due to its delicate strategic position between East and West, which made it the 'prepper nation of the Nordics' (Andersson and Pryser Libell, 2020). In spite of internal divides in society, the Swedes were in return keen to support their own choices, which allowed them to keep society more open and relied more on voluntary compliance with recommendations (Zølck, 2020). Hence the debate was not just about which country was best prepared or had the best health care, it was also about the meaning of universal welfare as a key Nordic value compared to the respect for democratic procedures and civil liberties.

Defending the Swedish line on multiple fronts

Over time, the Swedish model discourse has developed a tendency to become more blurred, aggregating too many diverse elements, relying on stereotypes, and it has become a target of information distortion and fake news. Because there has always been a great gap between this international reputation and the actual level of knowledge of the country or even the capacity for fact-checking, it is not so difficult to twist reality one way or another to show, for example, that certain things happen in Sweden that were previously unthinkable, such as urban riots and extreme violence. Even if this is not a radically new phenomenon, Paul Rapacioli argues that it took on a new dimension after the so-called 2015 immigration crisis and specifically in relation with this sort of sensitive issue that could be mobilized in other contexts, such as the debate on Brexit and immigration (Rapacioli, 2018b, p 84). National-populist politicians like Nigel Farage or Donald Trump have used this sort of rhetoric on several occasions and contributed to a diffusion of alternative, distorted visions of Sweden for the sake of their own political strategies.

Despite these trends in the representation of Sweden, there is no historical instance of such widespread and concentrated criticism of a public policy in Sweden as we have seen since 2020. There are of course memories of the past that were used to show that something was rotten in the kingdom, such as its compliance with Nazi Germany in World War II or its long-lasting experience of sterilization since the 1930s. The debate on a Swedish 'middle way' initiated by Marquis W. Childs back in the 1930s and whether it was only a light form of socialism not compatible with liberalism surfaced periodically until the 1970s and opposed various ideological streams, particularly in the US. More recently, debates have revolved around the nature and extent of change in a regime once praised for its uniquely egalitarian and redistributive profile and around the historical part social democracy played in this respect.[5]

This background is important to understand the representations of Sweden and Swedish values that influenced foreign expectations and judgements of the policies carried out in response to the pandemic. But they in turn informed many of the justifications raised by local actors – whether experts or politicians – or opinions circulated in the media in defence of the Swedish approach in a context of crisis (Simons, 2020, p 2). The deep polarization that ensued developed into a form of 'health care nationalism' that made it more difficult to express dissent at the domestic level and to question the choices made or the personal role and positions of certain key actors. This pandemic crisis was certainly a struggle against a new virus, but it was equally a trench war in terms of communication. In this respect, nowhere else was a public health agency and its representatives so much compelled to justify their actions not only to Swedish citizens but also to the rest of the world. Because Sweden prides itself on its long-standing and advanced principles or public transparency and is also very keen to monitor and preserve its favourable international reputation, the crisis has represented an extraordinary challenge. Given the nature and uncertainty of the pandemic, scientific experts of all disciplines and nationalities participated actively in the larger mediasphere, raising the level of knowledge and technicality in the debate while blurring the boundaries. However, it did not necessarily mean that expert positions had a stronger impact, probably because so much disagreement and so many contradictions were exposed.

Early justifications of the Swedish policies

From the beginning of the pandemic, the guiding principles as stated by the government in official discourse did not change substantially. The primary objective was to 'reduce the spread of infection' and 'flatten the curve' to 'safeguard human lives and secure a good health care capacity', 'reduce the impact on citizens and businesses' with 'appropriate measures at the right moment' that should also be weighted against their overall impact on society and public health. It was also stressed that each and every person should feel responsible and that it was important to provide access to reliable information in order to reduce anxiety and maintain a high level of trust in public authorities during a crisis that might last a long time.[6] Early on it was stated that the normal division of work, with FHM on the front lines to issue recommendations, would prevail, whereas political leadership was much more firmly asserted in the other Nordic countries. Answering the question of who is calling the shots in a press conference on 10 March, the Swedish health minister, Lena Hallengren, made it very clear that the government was following expert advice and would continue to do so.[7] Prime Minister Löfven repeated this in the parliamentary questions session on 17 March. All along citizens were urged to follow recommendations, stay home at the sign of any symptom, and wash hands and avoid crowded places. Besides, the Swedish law on communicable disease places responsibility on individuals to prevent spreading infection. People were also warned to beware of misinformation. Interestingly enough, while foreign countries often viewed the Swedish approach through the lens of exceptionalism – whether as good or bad – the Swedes insisted in the first place that their response was fully in line with their crisis procedures and that strict lockdowns with border closings would indeed mark a much sharper deviation from standard experience and expectations in a pandemic.

From the official experts' side, communication always took place in a matter-of-fact style, without resorting to dramatic effects or warlike rhetoric. One mantra was that recommendations and decisions should not be hasty but should be grounded in scientific evidence, which was obviously limited at the time. Yet because the tone was much less alarming than in many other countries, including the nearest neighbours, it could also be interpreted not only as underestimating the risk but also as sending the wrong signal to all that listened to FHM and relied on its recommendations for action, as Swedish epidemiologist Björn Olsen said in a TV debate on 26 February 2020. The direct response from the agency was that it was extremely difficult to find the right measure when a great majority of cases seemed to be mild and a small number of patients – mostly old and frail – ended up with complications and a lethal risk. The objective was to convey a message based on facts and not on fear and to promote 'a rational management' of the situation.[8] Public actors readily admitted that they did not know what was going to happen and urged taking it one step at a time even when other countries took more drastic measures. On the other hand, some experts seemed very determined in their rejection of the policies implemented elsewhere, such as border and school closures or lockdown. This attitude was quickly perceived as bordering on arrogance and stubbornness in the rest of the world, and it did not do any good to the Swedish reputation.

Even before controversies over mask mandates really took off, the fact that Sweden could keep restaurants, bars (as well as ski resorts) and schools open was the main source of debate. It should be noted that not all these venues actually remained open and that ski resorts closed at the end of March at the decision of the operators themselves. Due to advice to avoid overcrowding, attendance dropped naturally in public venues, and transportation as measured through mobile phone apps was on a par with other Nordic countries (Sulyok and Walker, 2021). As for schools, the recommendation was in favour of remote learning for high school, university and adult education. Yet comparisons often neglected the fact that Swedish schools are not as densely populated as, say, French or UK ones. The average number of pupils per class in primary school is currently under 20 versus almost 23 in France and up to 27 in the UK. Even in Sweden, it seems that the impact of COVID-19 also reduced the number of pupils attending school on a daily basis.

Ironically, Swedish state epidemiologist Anders Tegnell had co-authored a scientific article in 2009 with British epidemiologist Neil Ferguson on the effect of school closure, in the context of the swine flu episode. The publication aimed for a 'holistic perspective' with which to evaluate the multiple effects of such a measure, not simply the short-term reduction of infections: 'Health officials taking the decision to close schools must weigh the potential health benefits of reducing transmission and thus case numbers against high economic and social costs, difficult ethical issues, and the possible disruption of key services such as health care' (Cauchemez et al, 2009, p 1). This is what Swedes said they were doing all along, arguing that essential health workers had young children and anticipating the potential long-term effects not only of a psychological nature but also in terms of rising educational and social inequalities. On several occasions, Tegnell stressed the fact that all parents and children did not enjoy the same resources to ensure that proper education could be carried out remotely, and to work from home. But his correspondence later revealed that the measure could also be interpreted as aiming for the side-effect of herd immunity, when he wrote to his Finnish counterpart Mika Salminen as early as 13–14 March 2020 that children would spread the virus 'probably mostly to each other because of the extremely age-stratified contact structure we have' (Shilton, 2020). Retrospectively, most of the justifications advanced by the Swedish experts appeared to be tainted by this controversy on herd immunity as if they had conducted an experiment on the population, and one that failed cruelly.

More generally, the arguments against lockdown in Sweden were multiple. They ranged from the lack of legal and constitutional provisions to the absence of scientific evidence to back up this kind of drastic strategy. In other instances, Tegnell compared it to using a 'hammer to kill a fly', although the fly metaphor might not have been the most appropriate in retrospect. FHM also considered that they encouraged remote work early on in the impacted areas and that their recommendations had indeed modified the Swedes' lifestyle enormously (Milne, 2020). According to Tegnell, once visits to old-age homes were stopped as of 1 April 2020, locking down would not have prevented the high mortality in this sector, which accounted for nearly half of the casualties during the first wave (Osborne, 2020). The idea of sustainability was also put forward, as it seemed very difficult and detrimental to the social compact to impose stop-and-go policies over a long period of time that would most likely postpone infections, bring heavy social and economic distress, and ultimately meet opposition. Societies around the word – even democratic ones – have proven more resilient than expected in this regard, but even if Swedes did not anticipate that vaccines would come so fast, they were at least right in their belief that the pandemic would resemble a marathon race.

Sweden also distinguished itself in its refusal of any mask mandate in 2020, recommending wearing special gear only in the context of close contact with sick patients in hospitals. Masks were said to be used improperly by the general public and to give a false sense of protection that would undermine social distancing. However, the initial lack of supplies and the underestimation of asymptomatic cases certainly contributed to suboptimal protection in hospitals and nursing homes. The Swedish experts argued that they were following WHO guidelines in this respect. And it is true that, until June 2020, the organization did not make a strong case for masks apart for situations of close contact with symptomatic COVID-19 patients.[9] It then advised their use only in crowded environments, for all health care workers in clinical areas of a health facility, including those dealing with patients with COVID-19 and with people with vulnerabilities or over 60. But on this occasion WHO's General Director Tedros Adhanom Ghebreyesus nevertheless stressed: "I cannot say this clearly enough: masks alone will not protect you from COVID-19."[10] This is when Sweden started to distance itself from WHO guidance on masks, even if it was not more than a recommendation. But for a country that has always been a keen supporter of international organizations, it was still important to get some credit from the WHO, as that forms part of Sweden's reputation as a 'moral player' in world politics. In late February, Health Minister Lena Hallengren and International Development Minister Peter Eriksson held a press conference with the WHO director, who had himself studied in Sweden for a time, announcing extra financial support to the organization's crisis fund to support vulnerable countries.[11] This was not the most likely encounter that other European governments apart from the Nordic ones would have prioritized at the time. On several occasions, WHO representatives said that the Swedish approach should not be dismissed too quickly, as it trusted society to implement social distancing. In a late April 2020 press conference, Dr Mike Ryan, director of the health emergencies programme, commented:

> 'If we are to reach a new normal in many ways Sweden represents a future model of, if we wish to get back to a society in which we don't have lock-downs then society may need to adapt for a medium or potentially a longer period of time in which our physical and social relationships with each other will have to be modulated by the presence of the virus.'[12]

There was a gradual change in the Swedish official discourse during spring 2020 from the promotion of an alternative, liberal and sustainable strategy for fighting the pandemic to a much more defensive line that sought to minimize damage to its international reputation by any means (Simons, 2020, p 10). As soon as the UK changed tack, Sweden became more isolated (in the awkward company of Belarus) in Europe. With much higher infection and mortality rates than its neighbours and the controversies around herd immunity, the Swedish exception was viewed more negatively, except in the eyes of some conservative and libertarian streams that still hailed its respect for individual freedom and responsibility. But the latter tended to forget the role of the welfare state, with its significant health care capacity and comparatively generous compensation for the reduction of economic activity (Nguyen, 2020). In the meantime, the open records law in Sweden permitted access to a number of internal documents, mostly from FHM, that shed light on the internal discussions that shaped the official line and exposed some of the contradictions of the public discourse (Eriksson et al, 2020). Indeed, while denying that herd immunity was more than a potential side-effect, Swedish public authorities and experts maintained an ambivalent stance on this issue. Even if the rates of immunity in Stockholm proved 'disappointingly' low in June, the decline in virus circulation still raised hopes that the strategy might pay off after all (Mai, 2020).

Between herd immunity and health care nationalism

From April 2020 on, the debates started to revolve mostly around the hot potato of herd immunity and whether or not Sweden was playing with fire in this respect. This was also the time when opposition started to mount at home, especially within the scientific and medical milieu. Some had expressed concern or even dissent about the preparedness and strategy of the country early on, such as epidemiologist Björn Olssen, and even in the mainstream media, *Dagens Nyheter* Editor Peter Wolodarski had called for a lockdown at the start of March, criticizing the slowness and dubious assumptions of the Swedish response and urging a more decisive political lead in the crisis (Wolodarski, 2020a; 2020b). These were still isolated voices in a situation calling for a national consensus that is usually quite strong in Sweden, but they coalesced into a couple of visible initiatives that gathered mostly scientific personalities to plead with the government to step in as a result of the failure of the public health agency's strategy (Dagens Nyheter, 2020a). All this is now well documented: the groups stressed the underestimation of early warning signs and foreign experiences, the lack of anticipation that led to mortality rates on a par with worst-hit countries and created a climate of distrust at home.

In one of the articles, 22 researchers urged stricter measures to close public venues and impose family quarantines. But they also made a rare personal attack on the 'talentless civil servants' in charge of the response, which stirred up a lot of resentment.[13] Anders Tegnell and FHM were mostly dismissive of the criticism, arguing that the authors got their statistics wrong. They also responded that several countries that implemented strict lockdowns, such as Belgium, France and Spain, were even worse off. But it was clear from then on that there would be no real scientific debate between FHM and other experts. Later in May, in a rare expression of dissent among public servants, Tegnell's predecessor, Annika Linde, voiced criticism of FHM in a foreign media outlet, the UK's *Observer*, saying that shutting down earlier on would have bought time to protect the vulnerable (Orange, 2020b).[14] In spite of the common view that Swedish mainstream media outlets allow for a narrow range of opinions – commonly referred to as the 'opinion corridor' – this crisis has polarized it probably more than ever and will certainly leave scars (Andersson and Aylott, 2020 p 8).

In this debate, some of the positions adopted by experts at FHM, and particularly by senior epidemiologist Johan Giesecke, were considered much too self-assured – even arrogant – in a situation of high uncertainty, attracting rare criticism from the Norwegian public health authorities (Falkirk, 2020). In a few instances, Giesecke appeared confident in his predictions that lockdown would only delay infections and that mortality rates would even out between countries. His opinion was that most other countries were wrong and that democracies in particular would not accept such restrictions of basic freedoms for long. In addition, he seemed to be strongly convinced that the region of Stockholm that was the hardest hit would benefit from a significant degree of immunity at the end of the first wave, something that was not confirmed when antibody tests were performed (Giesecke, 2020). In tandem with Anders Tegnell, he created an image that, from outside, could be seen as a stereotype of Nordic coldness in facing the death toll of a pandemic, whereas it was more positively associated with pragmatism and sangfroid, even downright 'Swedishness', at home (Liljestrand, 2020). After his first appearances, Giesecke more or less disappeared from the media scene, and Tegnell remained the main expert communicating alongside the government in what increasingly resembled a competition between states and nations for the best strategy and a trench war of statistics. One good example was when Sweden was said to have reached the world's highest per capita mortality in April, measured over just a couple of days.

In early March FHM had triggered a small diplomatic crisis with Italy when Tegnell said that the Swedish health care system should be better equipped than its Italian counterpart to take the pandemic's first blow. In response, the Italian ambassador to Sweden felt compelled to reply that 'the struggle against COVID-19 is not a football game … it is a joint historical effort to safeguard the health of all people'.[15] With the Swedish strategy on trial in the spring, a political and diplomatic mobilization came about to better communicate and salvage the Swedish reputation and interests abroad. At the end of May, Foreign Minister Ann Linde had a virtual meeting with Swedish ambassadors, stressing that the national strategy had mostly the same goals and objectives for reduction of viral circulation and that it did not pursue any form of 'herd immunity' whatsoever (Lindberg, 2020a). This counter-offensive was all the more needed to prevent Sweden from being associated with the not-so-progressive regimes of Bolsonaro's Brazil, Nicaragua or Belarus.

Beyond this diplomatic mobilization to rescue the valuable Swedish brand, there was another kind of unexpected social activism to support soldier Tegnell and the lighter-touch approach promoted by the authorities. This movement triggered by both foreign and domestic criticism was termed 'public health nationalism' by some commentators and was the symptom of unprecedented polarization within Swedish society (Ahlström, 2020; Eriksson, 2020a). It was not so much an expression of partisan division, since most parties held ranks and refrained from strong criticism of the government. In contrast to many other countries, it was the nationalist SD Party that was the staunchest advocate of more stringent measures. But in the context of Swedish politics, this rising opposition force had been fighting to be included in an alternative political coalition. As it also supported better elder care and garnered support in the older generations, it was understandable that it stood up to protest when so many old people died in nursing homes.

However, expressions of patriotism were much more widespread and politically diffuse during the crisis. This was particularly attuned to a form of Swedish liberal or democratic nationalism (Gustavsson and Miller, 2019) that revolves around such values as trust, transparency, equality and rationality among others. As historian Lars Trägårdh has argued on many occasions, high reciprocal trust between government, experts and citizens is a key ingredient reflecting the kind of 'statist individualism' that he considers to be so specific to the Swedish social fabric. In addition, 'in a society where gender equality and children's rights are paramount', lockdown and school closure were very sensitive issues (Trägårdh and Özkirmli, 2020). As progressive as this might sound, this sociocultural analysis collided with another vision of progressiveness putting forward the protection of the frail and elderly who were the primary victims of the pandemic, thus questioning the real universality of the welfare system. These were opposite narratives and framings of the crisis that emphasized different, yet important dimensions of the Swedish democratic and welfare model imagery.

Finally, the most unexpected phenomenon in this crisis was certainly that all this tension should crystallize around the person of a previously unknown bureaucratic expert who held a press conference nearly every day at 2pm to comment on infection rates and repeat the same recommendations to wash hands and stay home at the sign of any symptom. To the utmost surprise of the man himself, Tegnell's face was not only printed on T-shirts but tattooed on forearms, while a Facebook fan-club page was set up with the following target: 'For all sensible people who believe it is better to act rationally on the basis of research instead of "forcefully" and in a populist fashion.'[16] Yet Tegnell also became the target of hate mail and threats, in a rare display of all the passions that such a crisis could stir. While he was keen to remind everyone that he was not even the chief of FHM and its 500 employees and was mostly issuing recommendations to the government and citizens, others pointed to the memory of social engineering revived by the present role of state expertise in the pandemic (Wiman, 2020), as if the agency had conducted some kind of experiment on Swedish society.

FOUR

Riding the Waves: Reckoning and Strategic Adjustments

By summer 2020, the first wave of COVID-19 in Sweden seemed to have run its course. The rate of new infections was finally on the way down, but the absolute death toll – over 5,000 already – appeared appalling. It was more than tenfold that of the other Nordic countries and, measured per capita, Sweden ranked among the 20 worst-off countries in the world. However, it should be remembered that each country had its own way of measuring fatalities; Swedish statistics compiled by FHM, for instance, count the number of persons who die with COVID-19 after PCR test confirmation, regardless of the actual cause of death (Garcia, 2021). In any case, the toll was very high, and nearly half of the mortality had been among those receiving elderly care. Whereas in the UK many elderly patients were in spring 2020 discharged from NHS facilities to nursing homes without even being tested (Amnesty International, 2020), in Sweden hard priorities were set, and many old people died in their residences without being transferred to ICUs, although the authorities claimed that there was no shortage of such emergency beds. The controversy triggered an inquiry by the Health and Social Care Inspectorate (Inspektionen för vård och omsorg, IVO) to establish whether people had been denied legitimate care. In June 2020, the military field hospital that had been set up in Stockholm was discontinued without having been put to much use. Facing the facts, the government was forced to admit that at least this essential objective of protecting the frail and elderly was a failure, although it was considered too early to judge the overall strategy. But from opposition leaders came words stronger than 'failure'. The leader of the SD, Jimmie Åkesson, called it a 'massacre'.[1] All this led the government to set up a commission of inquiry (Coronakommissionen) in June 2020 that would deliver its first, preliminary report in the autumn.

On the economic side of things, a small export-oriented economy was bound to suffer from the drastic reduction of activity worldwide, but it was hoped that the light-touch strategy would be less detrimental to the Swedish economy. In the first half of 2020, GDP had fallen by some 4%, much less than in France or the UK, but not so different from the other Nordic nations, which already had lower unemployment. At the same time, Sweden did not have to spend nearly as much in compensation as did countries that went into lockdown, and economic agents as well as consumers enjoyed higher stability and also less uncertainty (Persson and Sjöholm, 2021). In any case, the jury was still out because direct benefits did not appear outstanding and were subject to various appreciations (Bricco et al, 2020). Because of their new reputation as 'reservoirs' for the virus, Swedish travellers were still banned from neighbouring countries and many other destinations during summertime. It was also feared that misrepresentations and negative images of the country's strategy would hurt Swedish interests abroad. Yet, despite the high death toll, there was no sense of a social trauma, and levels of trust in the response to the pandemic remained high (Helsingen et al, 2020).

On multiple occasions state epidemiologist Anders Tegnell expressed his satisfaction with a strategy that seemed to have tamed the virus and gave hope that only isolated flare-ups would take place in the autumn. The idea that at least the capital region of Stockholm had gained some natural immunity one way or another was still in the air.[2] Around summer 2020, the Swedish experiment was slowly but surely becoming popular again in the big comparison game between nations, but internationally it was still segments of the Right that more fondly hailed the country led by a social democratic government. It was particularly so in Britain, where debate raged – even within Boris Johnson's party – over the continuation of emergency powers and the necessity to brace up for further lockdown as a result of increased circulation. In this context, Anders Tegnell was one of the experts to have a hearing with the British prime minister, and Sweden was pictured as the exemplar of those opposing new restrictions. Later on, in October, the Swedish case was indirectly featured again by an international anti-lockdown coalition of scientists and practitioners that launched the so-called 'Great Barrington Declaration', urging a more focused strategy in the pandemic.

The second wave eventually hit Sweden in the last months of 2020, and it did not spare the country as much as expected. At first, it triggered a slightly stronger political response, with new restrictions that were portrayed as the final verdict on the Swedish strategy in foreign media. Both the prime minister and the Swedish king were caught apologizing for the failure to protect the population more adequately. New pandemic legislation was even submitted to parliament and voted on in January 2021, in order to give more weight to the government. However, things did not change drastically through the next waves. Increased testing revealed more cases, and the death toll continued to deviate sharply from the rest of the Nordic region: throughout 2021, it was still nearly ten times that of Norway and Finland per capita and between three and four times that of Denmark, but it stood out less markedly in international comparisons. However, it continued to have a heavy bearing on relations with the neighbours. In 2021, the Swedish vaccination strategy did not differ much from the rest of Europe's: it took off at a slow pace and with the typical amount of debate, but it allowed Sweden to reclaim some of its moral leadership by fostering a more equal distribution of doses across the world. All the while most of the key actors remained on stage with a rather stable division of work between politics and expertise, until the prime minister decided to step down in autumn 2021. Nevertheless, the degree of polarization on home ground remained unprecedented.

This chapter will not aim for a detailed chronicle of a crisis that is still unfolding as I am writing these lines and is likely to impact our lives for quite some time. It will show that the role and representations of Sweden in the international discussion on pandemic responses remained significant for the better part of 2020, even if they were somewhat toned down in 2021 when vaccination became the core issue. To a large extent they continued to use the tropes of exceptionalism while still upsetting the traditional patterns of political support for the Swedish model. All along, a new form of health care diplomacy was deployed to minimize the negative impact on Swedish reputation and interests abroad, but also to promote a 'Swedish way' of dealing with the virus, with an ambivalent role played by state epidemiologist Anders Tegnell in this respect. Domestic conflicts persisted but were also mediated by the high level of transparency in public matters and ongoing inquiries into responsibility. In terms of policy, the overall stability should lend further support to the fact that a search for natural herd immunity was not the principal factor underlying the Swedish approach in the longer run. There were indeed important legal and practical adjustments to the policies and legal framework, but recommendations and trust continued to play a key role, while elementary schools and businesses remained open. Incentives to wear masks also slowly increased but remained limited in practice. The special inquiry was set up early on and helped to cast light on the distribution of responsibility, triggering a legitimate debate on crisis governance and elderly care reforms in particular and on the political and welfare system more generally.

A temporary return to grace for Sweden

The summer to early autumn of 2020 was a strange time for Sweden. After the country had been treated as a near pariah state, even by adjoining nations that did not open their borders to Swedish tourists, foreign discourse and representations started to shift again. COVID-19 infections and fatalities declined considerably and reached an all-time low in early September (see Figure 1), whereas they were growing again in countries that had ended their lockdowns in the spring. This was in line with what Swedish experts had forecast, that lockdown would only postpone flare-ups and pose a constant and painstaking dilemma of when and how to close down or open up. Could a country like France, the leading tourist destination in the world, afford to keep borders, restaurants and historical sites closed all summer? Although they reopened cautiously, much was at stake after months of lockdown and controls. The UK also slowly lifted restrictions and quarantines in July under the pressure of an economic slump of historic proportions. Yet signs of increased virus circulation were already showing up in July, although everyone wanted to believe that the virus would go away. In Sweden, despite the rather poor results of antibody testing, the idea was still in the air that the population had somehow managed to build up a degree of immunity and that occasional clusters would be limited. At the same time, Swedish experts believed that this virus was likely to stay around for a long time and that it was important to find a sustainable strategy supported by a majority.

After the WHO had also issued a severe judgment on virus circulation in Sweden at the end of June, the Swedish authorities reacted strongly and the WHO backtracked, stating that 'Sweden has involved the community in the response, and has been able to keep transmission to levels that can be managed by the Swedish health system' (Liman and Rolander, 2020). Later in the autumn, the WHO would update its recommendations in favour of avoiding prolonged lockdowns. Swedish travellers were still banned from a majority of places, but the country seemed to slowly regain some of its reputation. The diplomatic efforts to give a more nuanced image of the Swedish policies finally paid off.[3]

Figure 1: Daily new confirmed COVID-19 cases, March–September 2020

Shown is the rolling 7-day average. The number of confirmed cases is lower than the number of actual cases; the main reason for that is limited testing.

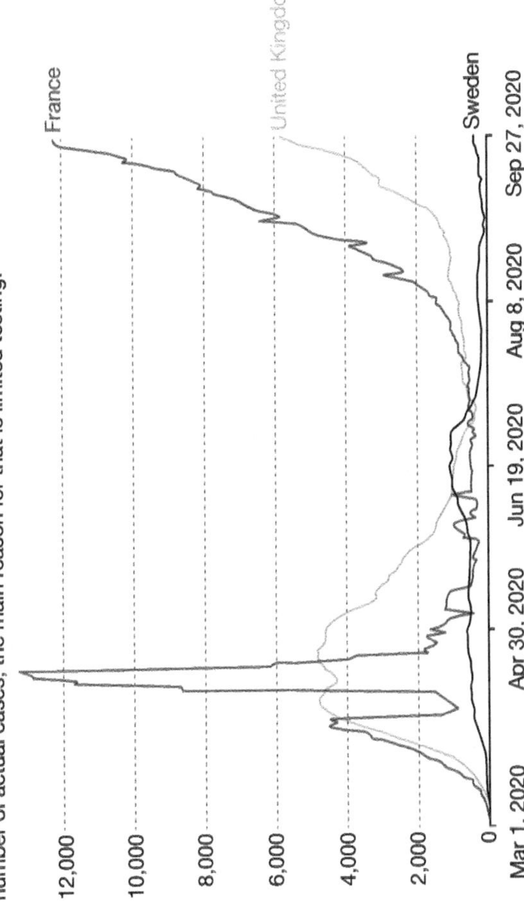

Source: Johns Hopkins University – retrieved from https://ourworldindata.org/covid-cases

The Swedish connection was particularly strong in the British scientific and political debate over the benefits of lockdown and the need to prepare for another one in case of a new epidemic surge. Newspapers such as the *Daily Telegraph* had for a long time welcomed the Swedish options (Clark, 2020; Woolhouse, 2020). Others, such as *The Sun*, which had remained mostly critical, started to change tone, publishing more positive coverage, as well as a portrait of Tegnell as a 'national hero' (Harvey, 2020). Another tabloid, the *Daily Mail*, was also more favourable, and it was not the least of paradoxes to find so many supporters of social democratic Sweden on the Right of the political spectrum, especially in the UK, whereas the Left was still more critical.

Indeed, other media more cautious about the Swedish approach, such as *The Guardian*, kept warning that the British welfare state and NHS were not even close to the Swedish system in terms of performance and benefit levels for loss of income or jobs. They pointed to the simplifications of a conflict between lockdowners and libertarians, with Sweden wrongly depicted as being representative of the latter grouping. If the Nordic country did not impose a lot of restrictions, it recommended a form of social distancing that – if respected – came down to a form of self-confinement for the many (Cohen, 2020).

Interestingly enough, Swedish experts started to play a more direct role in the British and international deliberation about which policy to adopt in case of a second wave. In the spring, Neil Ferguson and the Imperial College modelling had been decisive in triggering a change in the UK and elsewhere, in spite of the Swedish warning of the many biases in this alarming report. Ferguson was then blamed for his dire predictions and he would later be rebaptized 'professor lockdown' or 'doomster in chief'. This time around, it seemed that the UK government was ready to listen to different opinions, and Anders Tegnell was one of the experts briefing Boris Johnson and Chancellor Rishi Sunak after the prime minister had announced only limited restrictions, such as bar and restaurant curfews, at the end of September 2020. Earlier on, the UK Scientific Advisory Group for Emergencies (SAGE) had advised a short 'circuit-breaker' lockdown to prevent a new epidemic wave, and it appeared that meeting with Tegnell along with other scientists was influential in the decision to abstain (Sample, 2020).[4] It was around the same time that infections seemed to be on the rise again in Sweden, although it was not yet clear whether it could be attributed to more testing.

In the US, the Republican senator Rand Paul also referred to the Swedish open school policy during a conflict-filled hearing at which public health expert Anthony Fauci testified at the end of September (Edwards, 2020). On 4 October, a group of scientists led by two epidemiologists and one public health specialist from the UK and the US launched an initiative called the 'Great Barrington Declaration'. Sunetra Gupta (Oxford University), Martin Kulldorf (Harvard Medical School) and Jay Batthacharya (Stanford University) were the movers behind this declaration stating that 'Current lockdown policies are producing devastating effects on short and long-term public health', and that keeping lockdown measures in place 'until a vaccine is available will cause irreparable damage, with the underprivileged disproportionately harmed'. They advised a more 'focused' policy to protect vulnerable people while entirely reopening the sectors and activities that had been closed. At first glance it seemed to be a much clearer stance in favour of reaching herd immunity naturally, one that went beyond what Sweden had been doing, and it was severely attacked for being utterly reckless. Some Swedish scientists, such as epidemiologist Jonas Ludvigsson, nevertheless signed it, as did several thousand scientists around the world. Ludvigsson explained that he saw it from the global perspective of poorer countries, where the consequences of a reproduction of such drastic measures – and of the confinements in richer countries – would eventually cause more harm than the virus itself.

While Great Barrington was not in itself an explicit promotion of the Swedish approach, its idea of 'focused protection' could appear to share some similarities with what Sweden intended but failed to do in the beginning, that is to protect the old and frail while trying to mitigate the overall effects of the pandemic in society. On paper, it also claimed to adopt a more 'holistic' perspective on the consequences of the disease and of the policies, taking into account the health-related and socioeconomic impact of lockdowns that would – like the epidemic itself – add to the burden of the underclass. The initial support it received from a Trump presidency that was desperately seeking some scientific backing for its erratic response to the pandemic did not do the declaration any good. It was also endorsed by a large libertarian organization in the US, the American Institute for Economic Research. Sunetra Gupta was also one of the experts Boris Johnson consulted for policy guidance. And people like Brexit Party leader Nigel Farage also made mention of both Sweden and Great Barrington in their opposition to lockdowns in autumn 2020 (Kennedy, 2020).

As we can see, globally there were few voices from the Left and progressive circles that expressed clear public support for Swedish policies at the time, whereas the political patterns of support were much more mixed on home ground, with part of the Right and nationalists in opposition usually more critical. This political map was certainly another bewildering thing both for Swedish opinion at large and for decision makers who had been used to be on the more progressive side of things in international politics and still believed that what they were doing did not fundamentally depart from traditional Swedish values. All of a sudden, Sweden was neither the democratic socialist darling lauded by the likes of Bernie Sanders nor the 'next supermodel' for public sector reformers that *The Economist* once touted. This change was also particularly evident in the growing tensions with the other Nordic countries, which had kept their borders mostly closed except for regular commuters. In the summer and autumn there were controversies between

Norway and Sweden, for instance about which Swedish regions received clearance from Norway. Anders Tegnell also came up with a theory that some of the excess mortality among the elderly could be due to a mild influenza season the year before in Sweden, as in the UK and Belgium, whereas it may have been stronger in Norway. But Tegnell's Norwegian counterpart, Frode Forland, did not agree with this claim, reiterating that Norway's earlier and more stringent response was the main factor of differentiation between the two countries (Lindgren et al, 2020).

The final demise of exceptionalism

After this short respite in the pandemic, Sweden faced a second wave of infections, just as many other countries had. The caseload was already growing slowly in September and surpassed the other Nordics again in October. However, because hospitalizations and deaths remained low, the rise could still be attributed to more testing. The climate started to change when the large university town of Uppsala near Stockholm announced a 'voluntary lockdown' at the end of October. Nothing closed entirely, but the authorities called on the population to avoid socializing and even using public transport whenever possible. This was the first step in a series of more stringent measures throughout November that included stricter recommendations in other regions, renewed restrictions on visits to nursing homes and also reducing the limit for public gatherings and events from 50 to just eight people, as well as a national ban on serving alcohol after 10pm.[5] Places that had been relatively spared in the first wave were now more concerned by flare-ups, and FHM was, once more, accused of a lack of anticipation.

A new pandemic legal order

In a press conference on 16 November, Prime Minister Löfven indeed stressed the fact that recommendations had lost effectiveness and that stricter regulations might be in order. He described the eight-person limit for public events as a restrictive policy without equivalent in modern times. He considered it as a "very sharp signal" of the "new norm" for the entire Swedish society that everyone should refrain from as many social activities as possible, even below the threshold of eight participants and in private contexts as well.[6] This time around, parliament and government seemed to be more prepared to act forcefully if necessary, but the legal instruments available were still limited, for instance, to target certain types of private activities. The validity of the special powers voted on in April 2020 had lapsed without being put to much use at all.

In parliament, most of the opposition parties asserted their willingness to cooperate, yet they also asked for more clarity on the medium-term strategy. The answer from the government was that the strategy had not changed, that there were only important and temporary adjustments due to the gravity of the situation, but that the overarching goals were still to mitigate the overall effects of the epidemic on health but also on the economy and society at large while providing sound information to reduce anxiety.

Discussion on the suitable legal framework for these extraordinary times was nevertheless in flux. In October the government announced that it would lay the ground for special and temporary pandemic legislation to be voted on, but the initiative was shared between the parliament's social affairs committee and the Centre Party. As some party leaders pointed out, eight months had elapsed since the beginning of the crisis and the government had not sought a more effective legal instrument to fight the pandemic. The prime minister's justification was that the extra powers voted in April had not been used, that the constitutional and parliamentary order called for specific review of this kind of important legal change that might infringe more severely upon civic liberties: "We have to make sure that the rate of infections is kept low ... but we also have to stand up for the basic values of our society."[7]

To hear a head of government say this in front of parliament several months into a crisis of this magnitude was particularly indicative of the difference that Sweden still cultivated in this crisis context. This is another example of the 'soft power' approach used by the Swedish government that stands in sharp contrast with the emergency and extraordinary powers that many other executives could rely on during the crisis (Cameron and Jonsson-Cornell, 2020).

When preparatory work started, the government counted on a new law to be in place only by spring or even summer 2022. In fact, it went through much faster than anyone expected, with a first version implemented on 10 January 2021, but not without resistance or worries. The special 'remiss' system in Sweden implies the widespread consultation of various institutions and sectors of society before a new policy or law is enacted. In her statement on the project, Chief Justice Ombudsman Elisabeth Rynning expressed her acknowledgment of a legal instrument that would allow the government to act more swiftly and forcefully with regard to the crisis situation, possibly at the expense of some basic freedoms, but she nevertheless voiced deep concern about the extensive delegation of power from the legislative to the executive branch, thus rejecting the proposal in its initial form. The timing and duration of this extraordinary legislation was also questioned with respect to its impact on civil liberties, economic activity and daily life (JO, 2020). The ombudsman would entertain similar misgivings in April 2021 when a four-month extension of the law was considered, as of September. Even the nationalist SD Party, which earlier had called for more powerful interventions, expressed concern about the risks that this pandemic law might hold for businesses and freedoms, that it could eventually lead to something like a soft lockdown (Bäckström Johansson, 2021). Eventually, all parties insisted on the necessary compensation provisions for losses that businesses and individuals should incur as a consequence of further restrictions, but this belonged to the budgetary discussion.

In international media, this evolution was essentially regarded as a U-turn and as final evidence of the failure of the Swedish light-touch approach, without any consideration for the actual democratic process that was going on. Along with new and more stringent restrictions and some voluntary local 'lockdowns', special pandemic legislation apparently pointed to more government control and added to the litany of failure acknowledgments pronounced by the prime minister and even the king of Sweden, Carl Gustaf, at the end of 2020 (Mann, 2020; Pancevski, 2020; Pieper, 2020). What foreign observers had misunderstood or failed to grasp, however, was the combined effect of several elements of the Swedish political order that made it very difficult to substantially reinforce the delegation of power to the executive in peacetime and impose anything close to a strict lockdown. Adjustments had to be made in a piecemeal fashion. In many other countries – even democratic ones – it could be pictured as a sign of weakness and failure to act. Yet, to a large extent, the Swedish executive managed the crisis in close cooperation with parliament, expert agencies and local government, which could lead to significant delays, coordination problems and even conflicts, but it was justified by domestic decision makers as standard constitutional and democratic procedure. Legal constraints were indeed substantially tightened during the winter, but it is debatable whether that amounted to a radical shift in approach. In other words, Sweden more or less pursued its strategy of mitigation, fine-tuning the balance between mandatory restrictions and recommendations in accordance with FHM. The official stance on face masks evolved somewhat, with the advice to wear them in public transport during rush hours in spring 2021; remaining public venues such as libraries or swimming pools had to close, and restrictions were tightened on restaurants' and bars' hours and alcohol service.[8] Fines could be levied for non-compliance, but controls remained moderate in a high-trust society.

Sweden in the global rush for vaccines

The real game changers in this crisis came earlier than expected – at the turn of 2021 – with several vaccine formulas marketed by Pfizer, Moderna and Astra Zeneca, mostly for the Western world, and others devised by China and Russia that reached parts of the southern hemisphere in a situation of global shortage. To a great extent, the arrival of vaccines modified the parameters of the crisis and of national strategies to battle COVID-19. Although it would take time to distribute them widely and appreciate their real-world effectiveness, they opened the possibility for large-scale prevention and immunity. At the time of writing, we were still in the early phase of this development that made Sweden look less different from other welfare states.

Swedes are indeed good disciples when it comes to vaccination, which is usually not mandatory, exhibiting up to 98% compliance for children. At the beginning of the 2009 swine flu epidemic, the public health authorities and Anders Tegnell recommended widespread vaccination, prompting 60% of the population to get the Pandemrix vaccine from GlaxoSmithKline. However, it occasioned some serious adverse effects in the form of narcolepsy, triggering compensation, and that somewhat undermined the generally high trust in these medical products in Sweden.[9] For COVID-19 vaccines, the proportion of the population that doubted them was high in the beginning, but there was little information available at the time. By March 2021, the rate of acceptance had jumped to almost 90% (Rolander, 2020; Folkhälsomyndigheten, 2021). The main question for Sweden was about securing contracts for vaccines, as some worried that the Swedish strategy so far would make it more difficult to strike a quick and fair deal with companies. There were also some initial controversies regarding the profile of the vaccine coordinator, Richard Bergström, who had formerly headed the European

Federation of Pharmaceutical Industries and Associations and was also a member of the EU negotiation team. There was a lack of transparency in vaccine negotiations at the national and European levels, which could be seen as an obstacle to building trust, but countries were desperate to get their share. Ultimately most of the debate revolved around the logistical challenge of rolling out vaccination throughout the regions that are responsible for health care in Sweden. It resulted in a relatively slow pace for the immunization campaign at first, in a context of global shortage and with added problems linked to Astra Zeneca delivery and safety. However, by the end of summer 2021, some 80% of the adult population had received one injection and 65% had undergone complete vaccination.

For a country like Sweden with a strong history of solidarity with more deprived countries, it was also expected that the question of global distribution and availability of doses would be of importance. Even representatives of the medical industry voiced concern early on about the risks of vaccine nationalism that might result in highly skewed access around the globe (Blanck, 2021). Sweden is one of the original six donor countries to the Global Alliance for Vaccines (GAVI) launched in 2000 by the Bill and Melinda Gates Foundation and has pledged an all-time high of SEK1.75 billion for the 2021–2025 period. It is also the world's largest per capita contributor to the Covax initiative for a more equitable distribution of vaccines.[10] In making these commitments, along with the direct donation of millions of non-earmarked doses, Swedes were back on a much more familiar terrain of international solidarity and global health that has greatly contributed to their favourable reputation abroad. As often before, this was not completely devoid of vested interests, Astra-Zeneca being a British–Swedish corporation, and through its partnership with the Serum Institute of India – the world's largest vaccine maker – the company planned for large-scale production of inexpensive doses that could compete with Chinese vaccines. At a Swedish–Indian virtual forum in

March 2021, Stefan Löfven praised India for being the new "pharmacy of the world",[11] though the dramatic surge of the virus's Delta variant in that spring made India less willing to ship doses abroad. In the deep crisis that ensued, the Swedish Chamber of Commerce called on businesses in India to mobilize in partnership with diplomatic services and NGOs in order to provide urgent aid.[12] There were also limits to this global solidarity, as Swedish vaccine coordinator Richard Bergström said, with a priority to vaccinate teenagers while coverage of vulnerable people in poor countries remained low (Von Hall, 2021).

As Sweden healed its wounds, there were signs that it was recovering some of its reputation as a global 'moral' player that had promoted the country's interests abroad in the past (Irwin, 2019). Swedish leaders and diplomats continually spread the message that their national choices in the crisis were not unfounded and that the consequences of the pandemic and responses to it, especially for poorer countries, went much beyond the tragic loss of so many lives. For instance, in his introductory speech to Sweden's voluntary national review on implementation of the 2030 Agenda at the United Nations, Prime Minister Löfven did just that when he stressed that "for many the pandemic has had far-reaching impacts ... global unemployment has increased and many families have seen their income drop. School closures have had damaging impact on many children ... . Poverty, inequalities and gender-based violence have increased".[13]

However, despite the country's support for vaccination in the Global South, it sometimes proved more difficult to reach foreign-born populations and minorities back home. These communities, more concentrated in suburban areas, had already paid a higher price in terms of casualties in 2020 and were occasionally pointed at for their particular role in the initial spread of coronavirus (Zangana, 2020). In truth, their health, living and working conditions made them more vulnerable to both the virus and the restrictions to fight it, and the United

Nations warned against this inequality (Collste, 2020).[14] In the vaccine rollout in 2021, foreign-born populations lagged behind for all age categories by a significant margin, with a strong income correlation (Folkhälsomyndigheten, 2020). It looked as if the solidarity that was demonstrated toward foreign countries in need of help reached its limits in relation to deprived communities at home.

Evaluating responsibility

As early as June 2020, a special commission of inquiry on the pandemic response was set up in Sweden. When something important and controversial occurs, it is customary in Sweden to appoint such a commission in order to defuse conflict, lay out responsibilities and make recommendations for future improvements. In this respect, Sweden again did not depart from standard procedures, although the government initially hoped to postpone the inquiry until after the crisis. When the commission was appointed, the parliamentary opposition insisted that it be independent from parliament. Since mainstream parties had been in relative agreement on the initial strategy, this arrangement was regarded as preferable, although separate commissions would later be named within parliament to scrutinize the actions of the political branch itself.

Public inquiries and the scandal of elderly care

This 'Corona Commission', as it was referred to, was headed by a former justice and head of the Supreme Administrative Court, Mats Melin. Apart from him, it included four women and three men, among them several academics from a variety of disciplines, a former director of the federation of local governments and a female priest. The first objective assigned to this organ was to carry out a systematic review of crisis management at all levels and of its effects. The work was done so effectively that the first report, focused on elderly care, was ready by December 2020. In addition, the IVO (the Health Care Inspectorate) and other organizations such as the municipal employees' unions had also commissioned separate reports on the matter that came in at about the same time.

As a result, even if the opposition parties still appealed to consensus and national solidarity, the tone of the debate became slightly more accusatory again by the end of 2020. The government was increasingly blamed for the belatedness and slowness of testing in the spring and for its alleged tendency to hide behind FHM or the regions. The different reports made the real distribution of the death toll starkly clear, although it was not breaking news. In his official presentation on 15 December 2020, the commission chairman Mats Melin noted that nine out of ten of the 7,000 people who had died of COVID-19 so far were over 70, one-quarter received some kind of home care and nearly one-half were living in nursing homes. This was a real pandemic of the frail elderly and striking evidence of a failure of a national strategy that claimed to be protecting them first of all.

The commission considered that the main responsibility lay with the government – and its predecessors – who were well aware of the structural problems in elderly care, even if other organizations participated in this collective failure, especially elderly care providers at the local level. By stressing the correlation between high circulation of the virus and mortality in nursing homes, the commission indirectly targeted the overarching approach laid out by FHM and implemented by political authorities. In light of this widespread circulation, the specific needs of nursing home residents and staff to protect themselves were not identified soon enough, tests were not carried out, the national ban on visits to these institutions came too late and it did not even accommodate the basic rights of families to say their last goodbyes. However, the report also emphasized structural difficulties in the old age care sector: unclear and fragmented responsibilities for service provision and a lack of staff and skills (especially medical), with a number of workers doing shifts in several institutions.[15] Norway, for instance, had a much higher number of nurses with a stable contract in care homes and was better equipped with medical staff (Huuponen, 2020). In addition to this already grim picture, IVO's own inquiry showed that a high number of old people in care facilities were left to suffer or die without medical consultation or adequate pain relief such as oxygen (IVO, 2020). Further inquiries, for example by Swedish public radio, showed that a number of families were not even informed of palliative measures administered to their relatives (Sadikovic and Ridderstedt, 2020). Because of the prioritization system at times of elevated pressure on hospitals, sick patients over a certain 'biological' age (with pathologies) and in nursing homes were rarely transferred and medical assessment was regularly done by telephone, or not at all. But IVO also stressed that priorities were sometimes unwarranted even in hospitals, where some patients could have been given better survival chances (Röstlund and Gustafsson, 2020). All the time, FHM boasted that ICU capacities never reached the point of saturation and field hospitals that were built, as in Stockholm, were hardly put to use. However, even if all the beds were not full, it does seem that specialist staffing was not sufficient to operate ICUs in acceptable conditions.

In October 2020, Amnesty International published a harsh report on the situation of nursing homes in the UK, with evidence that a significant number of older patients were discharged from hospitals into elderly care units in spring 2020 without prior testing and with the objective of preserving a strained NHS. Those patients contributed to the deadly wave of contaminations (Amnesty International, 2020). The judgment on Sweden was arguably less severe, but it was nevertheless unusual for this country to stick out so negatively in international comparisons. As journalist Björn Elmbrant pointed out, the prevalence of mortality among elderly people confined in care homes and among minorities living in poor suburban areas put a spotlight on a form of underclass in

Swedish society (Elmbrant, 2020). People in these categories lived in dwellings that were cornerstones of the postwar welfare state, care residences and mass housing complexes built in the 1960s in the peripheries of larger cities. The latter came to be increasingly populated by new immigrants who were, in turn, more likely to work in services such as elderly care. A 2013 report had already shown that one-quarter of employees in this sector were foreign born, and the proportion reached 50% in the Stockholm region, 30% of them with insecure contracts (Wondmeneh, 2013). These precarious employees, such as assistant nurses (*undersköterskor*),[16] many of them women, now represent Sweden's single largest professional category. They are economically more vulnerable, cannot work remotely, are more likely to have different workplaces and are more dependent on public transportation. Elderly care sector workers may have been poorly informed about the actual risks of infection at an early stage, but they were most likely facing a dilemma because their presence is also essential to the survival of care home residents in situations of chronic understaffing. A 2018 report of Sweden's Work Environment Authority reported that assistant nurses appeared to be twice as likely as other employees to go to work while sick (Berggren and Martinsson, 2018). In early April 2020 the municipal employees' union (Kommunal) actually tried to lobby in favour of wearing masks along with visors when in contact with suspected or confirmed COVID-19 patients. But the city of Stockholm disputed this; the Work Environment Authority initially sided with the union before surprisingly reversing its judgment after a meeting with the federation of local governments, the main provider of elderly care. The dispute was settled in court and did not support a straightforward policy in this matter (Bankel et al, 2020).

Learning the hard lessons

As we have seen, elderly and health care in Sweden are prerogatives of different levels of local government, from municipalities to regions, with a division of work that renders coordination difficult. The number of private providers of elderly care has also increased significantly in the last 20 years, adding new layers to this already complex picture. As a result of the pandemic, the decentralized but also fragmented governance of the Swedish welfare system has been severely criticized (IVO, 2020; Lindberg, 2020b). Neither the government nor the specialized agencies managed to provide an efficient implementation at the local level of some of the recommendations and policies that they produced. But the political branch and the expert agencies were not always in full agreement regarding the priorities of the day. The difficulties seen in kick-starting a more massive testing effort in April 2020 provide good evidence of the complex interplay between actors and their embedded interests and also of the typical rigidities of a highly procedural administrative and political system: in March 2020, parties in parliament put pressure on the government, which had problems coming to agreement with FHM and the regions about the perimeter and (financial) responsibilities for testing. On 8 May, Social and Health Care Minister Lena Hallengren held a press conference to announce the goal of 100,000 tests per week. She invited representatives of the regions but they did not even bother to show up, which gives an idea of the authority of ministers in Sweden. As a result, the government had to name a national coordinator for testing, Harriet Wallberg, and only in June did the capacity increase significantly.

In this context, political scientist Bo Rothstein argued that local self-government proved to be the real Achilles' heel in the crisis. He called for a substantial constitutional revision that would place it more clearly under the direct leadership of the executive in case of crisis, adding that political representatives should not hide behind expert agencies in situations of high uncertainty (Rothstein, 2020). Other observers rightly claimed that FHM's dual role in evaluating the epidemiological risk and making recommendations or policies based on a much wider appreciation of societal and even economic consequences was highly problematic (Wierup and Wågsholm, 2020). It could even be said that it created an anomaly, to judge from the extraordinary role that one single expert – Anders Tegnell – came to play in the public's eye, acting as the ultimate guarantor of Swedish policies, at home and abroad.

In December 2020, FHM responded to the reports and the high mortality in nursing homes by stating that it had early on made warnings and recommendations to protect the elderly and that the responsibility for running those facilities ultimately lay with local government. Yet because its recommendations basically left it to the determination of local employers – and not even employees – whether masks or other protections were useful, and because of a weak testing policy until late spring 2020, it was problematic to shift responsibility entirely, even though material supply was clearly a problem at the start of the epidemic. Indeed, local governments were left to interpret the hesitations on mask wearing, particularly in light of what other countries were doing, and service providers sometimes improvised protections (Keussen et al, 2020). There was a tendency on the part of FHM leadership and top experts to find other more 'external' explanations that might account at least in part for the high death toll in care homes, such as the light flu season in Sweden the previous year or the fragmented governance structure for crisis management and health care. But they certainly had a hard time acknowledging the direct effects of their own response and recommendations.

The Swedish system for establishing responsibility, identifying failures and making recommendations for improvements has its origins in a relatively consensual order that aims to defuse criticism, and it has been quite successful at that over time. The system of parliamentary commissions including representatives of the different parties has weakened considerably and has been replaced by special investigator's inquiries often led by bureaucrats (Dahlström et al, 2020). In addition, the political climate in Sweden has undoubtedly changed a lot over the last

20 years, accompanied by an increased radicalization of political debate. The COVID-19 crisis has led to a new degree of polarization in society, though the parties themselves managed to limit political conflict. Exposed personalities such as Anders Tegnell started to receive serious threats, even death threats, that prompted the authorities to grant him personal protection. In a society where elites pride themselves on behaving like everyone else, cycling to work or taking public transportation, in spite of the assassination of two high-profile political personalities in the last 35 years,[17] this is a telling indicator of the degree of change. On the other hand, there was no witch hunt as a result of COVID-19, and most of the actors remained in place. The only significant exception was the public repudiation of the director of MSB (the civil contingency agency), Dan Eliasson, who went on a discreet family trip to the Canary Islands over Christmas 2020 at a time when only essential travel was advised. He did not break any rules, in contrast with British political adviser Dominic Cummings or epidemiologist Neil Ferguson, who were caught in breach of UK's lockdown in 2020, but he nevertheless undermined the almost sanctified trust that Swedes supposedly place in their public servants and leaders; hence he probably served as a form of Christmas sin-offering for all the people who were stranded.

Although it will take time to carry out reforms of crisis governance as well as health and old age care, there are grounds to believe that the magnitude of the shock was given its due weight in Sweden, or at least more than in many other places. In countries such as the UK or France that experienced comparable mortality in care homes and even higher hospital saturation, public commissions have either been postponed or did not enjoy the same visibility. In the UK, Boris Johnson resisted such an inquiry and decided to put it off until 2022;[18] in France, both the national assembly and the senate delivered their first report at the end of 2021. They were broad and critical enough but have failed to trigger much public debate to date, even in a presidential election campaign. In France, the hospital crisis had been a widely discussed topic for a long time, on a par with the NHS in the UK, but elderly care was also in dire need of more attention and has not yet received it in proportion to the human losses incurred in the pandemic. I will return to this issue of social and health care institutions in relation to the larger welfare complex in the next chapter.

FIVE

Recasting the Swedish Model in Crisis Mode

The pandemic, and the policies devised in response, have had a profound but highly unequal impact on countries across the world, and it will take time to fully grasp the nature and extent of the implications. Battling COVID-19 and facing historic economic downturns in 2020, the most well-off nations resorted to public debt at a wartime scale. However, compensation schemes for job and activity losses and investment to boost the economy were uneven. Politicization of crisis management was stronger in some countries – such as the US, where the ascent to the presidency of Democrat Joe Biden changed federal government policies radically. Restrictions and mask or vaccine mandates tied to public health were tightened; structural investment and budgets of a magnitude unseen since World War II have been put forward by the Democratic administration. The government is advancing proposals to raise taxes on top incomes and make tax collection more effective. This is a major programmatic shift that is likely to have an impact beyond the US, although part of this ambition faces opposition.

Many other countries have witnessed considerable increase of public debt and a renewed role for the state and for health care or elderly care institutions, but it is not clear whether these will substantially change the politics of welfare and health care reforms that prevailed before the pandemic struck. In the UK and France, where hospitals and long-term care have been under pressure for a long time, plans have been announced or passed to raise taxes and sometimes wages. Recently, in September 2021, Boris Johnson broke Conservative vows with a proposal to impose a new flat tax of 1.25% to fund better care and make it more affordable, but also to 'rescue the NHS'. He also aimed to put a cap on lifetime individual expenses for elderly care. The proposal was immediately criticized as unfair and too narrow even to catch up with the huge backlog of untreated non-COVID-19 cases. Behind the scenes, it was not clear whether the bill sent to parliament in September 2021 would challenge competitive tendering and fragmentation within the NHS and re-establish more political control, or if it would lead to more deregulation. In France, the summer 2020 negotiations ended in wage hikes for health care workers and significant investment in elderly care, but it was not enough to compensate for the systemic lack of staff, underfunding and low pay in these fields as the long pandemic literally exhausted the medical and care professions.

Sweden fell somewhere in between the US and the UK or France, because it suffered a hard blow and the consequences in terms of mortality in particular made its long-praised welfare model look not just vulnerable but possibly guilty of serious negligence. Neoliberal inroads into the welfare and health care system have not gone as far as in the UK, but they nevertheless changed the picture profoundly, to the extent that universal and egalitarian commitments became less evident and that social democracy shed significant parts of its identity in the process (Kamali and Jönsson, 2018). In many ways, the pandemic laid bare some of the fault lines of the Swedish model that had long been known locally but remained somewhat concealed by a reputation of progressiveness and performance. In addition, the crisis carved out a divide within what could be regarded as a common Nordic model. Not only did Sweden distinguish itself markedly from the other Nordics, showing that coordination in hard times was not necessarily natural, but the pandemic also left traces of hard feelings between national communities, especially between Sweden and Norway.

Political representations of the Swedish model have been modified in the process. This is by no means the first time, in as much as this notion has proved flexible enough to integrate many different components and allowed for reinterpretations. By and large the property of the social democratic Left, the model started to evolve along with welfare and public sector reforms in the 1980s and 1990s toward a potentially interesting country case for other political families leaning to the Right, a development that prompted academic discussions as to the actual nature of this model in relation to contemporary capitalism (Lindbom, 2001; Bergh, 2013; Belfrage and Kallifatides, 2018).

Pensions but also health care and elderly care have been cornerstones of this transformation, with major reforms in the 1990s that created an increasingly decentralized, deregulated and fragmented system (Granberg et al, 2021). The pandemic shock placed the emphasis on particular sectors that deal with ageing and vulnerable populations. High mortality in care homes and coordination problems with primary and hospital care exposed some of the deficiencies of the Swedish welfare state. The recession also triggered renewed discussions about the problems of unemployment insurance, in spite of comparatively good levels of compensation for the loss of activity that were guaranteed as a result of this crisis. With the sudden decision of Prime Minister Löfven to quit rather than seek a new mandate as party leader in autumn 2021, this electoral year of 2022 may be an important test for the collective capacity to draw the right lessons in this new era.

The Swedish rebuttal of strict lockdown or mask mandates put the country on the map for political groups that are not usually fond of what the Swedish model stands for. British and North American conservatives and libertarians, accompanied by populists and nationalists of different kinds, rediscovered a Sweden that seemed to place civil liberties and responsibilities first, that kept primary schools, gyms, restaurants and bars open and claimed to mitigate the overall effects of the pandemic on society. By contrast, the moderate Left and Right that make up the bulk of traditional Swedish supporters kept their distance, criticizing the failure of an advanced welfare state to protect its vulnerable elderly population and to hold down the mortality rate on a par with its Nordic neighbours. These changing representations triggered diplomatic and public relations offensives to communicate that what Sweden was doing was not unique or plainly wrong. Yet, paradoxically, the pandemic also attracted unprecedented interest in the country, and not only negative interest. Sweden thus became a benchmark against which other national strategies that adopted more or less constraints were regularly compared, with important normative connotations. I have shown how this heated discussion mobilized experts, scientists and intellectuals as well as politicians, journalists, bloggers and the general public, mainly via the internet.

Indeed, the pandemic and its responses have raised essential philosophical and political questions about the vulnerability and value of human life, the price we are ready to pay for good health care and other care, the limits to emergency and exceptional procedures in times of crisis in order to safeguard democracy and civil liberties and the construction and role of scientific evidence and expertise (Landström, 2020). The Swedish case has been featured in these debates perhaps more ambiguously than ever before, as some sort of battlefield that also polarized opinion at home. Crises of this magnitude have the potential to be game changers, and some have described the pandemic as a 'total social fact' in the sense of anthropologist Marcel Mauss (Gaille and Terral, 2021), the kind of event that alters the life of everyone. Although Swedes allegedly enjoyed more freedom to go about their everyday lives, they were nevertheless unequally affected by the crisis, and they certainly felt the shock of being ostracized even in their own Nordic region.

Welfare responses

One important dimension that was surprisingly little discussed during the pandemic crisis was the diverse capacity and readiness of (welfare) states to compensate for some of the losses incurred in the historic slowdown of the economy and for the increased workload of certain professions, particularly in the health care sector. The focus on the immediate death toll apparently due to the virus and on the resources to reduce its impact made the consequences of this slowdown less visible, at least in countries where the state could afford to alleviate some of the material losses. In many parts of the world where informal work prevails or there is a high dependency on trade and tourism, the effects of the pandemic and global lockdowns were inevitably more direct and drastic and may be long-lasting. Since the first wave in 2020, there has been a tendency to bring this debate down to a rather crude trade-off between human fatalities, on the one hand, and economic buffering, on the other, with Sweden often featuring as the example of a morally but also economically wrong gamble. Observers were keen to point out the apparently limited financial gains that the avoidance of lockdown permitted (Goodman, 2020). Yet the overall cost of the pandemic will have to be calculated over several years, and protecting the economy and businesses was but one of the goals of the mitigation strategy chosen by Sweden. Larger social and psychological impacts, especially in the case of school closure, were also taken into account.

The objective here is not to provide any thorough review of the main policies to alleviate the effects of the pandemic on society but to argue that the crisis reframed some of the essential questions raised by welfare and health care reforms in the last three decades, casting new light on the capacity and role of the modern state in Sweden and beyond. Apart from rolling out vaccines and allocating historically large sums to local governments to increase health care capacity, Swedish lawmakers agreed to maintain liberal and generous compensation to relieve employers of extra costs related to sickness pay; they voted on special benefits for people at risk who could not carry out their work as usual (up to SEK80, about £7, per day) and for parents who had to care for young children when some schools or classes closed, raised housing benefits for families with children by 25% and improved support for single parents.[1] Waiting periods for receiving sickness pay and medical certifications were also removed early on, in order to make it easier for people with symptoms to stay at home from day one. Wait times for unemployment insurance were also suppressed, and qualifying conditions were relaxed (Greve et al, 2020).

However, all this did not make Sweden the promised land for people who lost their livelihoods. Because unemployment insurance there is voluntary and results from collective agreements, it has long been a target for its shrinking coverage and replacement rates. In 2021, Sweden ranked 21st in the OECD in this area, just above Greece, and last in the Nordic region. With the steep rise in unemployment during the pandemic, especially in certain sectors, the benefit level was slightly raised, and some unions demanded that increases be made permanent (Selnes, 2021). The situation gave new wind to the call from several parties (interestingly, mostly on the Right) for a tax-financed compulsory insurance, a position that the Left has been less inclined to support for fear that it would undermine union density and strength. This is an old bone of contention between parties that dates back to the belated and painful introduction of unemployment insurance in 1934 by the Social Democrats. It fuelled criticism because of the organic ties between the largest trade union federation, Landsorganisationen (LO), and the Social Democratic Party. These ties remain, though they have weakened over time, and a large membership is seen by the Right as a piggy bank for this party. The pandemic thus triggered a renewal of this long-standing debate that lies at the heart of the Swedish social democratic regime, leading the government to set up yet another public commission in August 2021 to investigate potential reforms of unemployment insurance schemes. This is one of the enduring paradoxes of a Swedish model usually conceived of in terms of universal coverage, but which is also made up of less secure and less encompassing institutional arrangements.

As far as employment is concerned, professionals in the health and home care sectors were naturally in a radically different situation, facing a historic increase of their workload, the need to drastically scale up medical and hospital capacity, and the requirement of testing and all the safety procedures to keep the virus at bay. For a Swedish welfare state that has considerably rationalized the hospital sector and deregulated elderly care to a large extent since the early 1990s, COVID-19 could be seen as a strong wake-up call. All of a sudden, the basic tenets of new public management that had so powerfully influenced reforms of the public welfare system were turned upside down: more staff, beds and equipment were needed, field hospitals had to be built in all haste in Stockholm and Gothenburg, patients were stranded in hospitals for long periods of time and better coordination between primary and specialized care as well as between local and national levels was on the agenda. Long before the pandemic, Sweden faced a deficit of health care professionals – especially nurses – and of hospital resources, and there were tensions surrounding wages and work conditions. Yet the Swedish system managed to ramp up its hospital and emergency care capacity significantly during the pandemic, at least in the most severely impacted urban areas.

It failed to achieve the same degree of national mobilization for elderly care, which is even more locally run and with uneven conditions. Yet it was not the case that elderly care had not been on the political agenda before. The Centre-Right government led by Fredrik Reinfeldt had started an inquiry in 2014 with a view to improving coordination between health and elderly care (Heldahl et al, 2020). The first Löfven government stopped it but invested significantly in housing and staffing after 2016. In addition, that government initiated a complete review of social service law in 2017, and Lena Hallengren, the present minister of health and social affairs who then held the portfolio of children and the elderly, gave instructions in 2018 to look into whether separate legislation was needed for old-age care.[2] The difficulties that plague this sector – part-time and hourly employment with an overrepresentation of low-skilled workers and geographical inequalities in the provision and quality of services – are well known. Municipal governments in charge have dedicated unequal resources to this growing sector and contracted out to a number of private providers, resulting in important variations in cost and quality (Stolt and Winblad, 2009). This situation is by no means limited to Sweden; countries like France or the UK face related problems, sometimes with even much higher user costs. Comparatively, the high mortality in care institutions seems to have made a stronger impact on Sweden. A program of paid education for low-skilled workers was funded by the state in May 2020, in agreement with local actors and unions. The 2021 budget included the highest endowment ever, at more than SEK7 billion, to municipalities to improve the state of elderly care. Although it is still unclear how local government and contractors will use this money and what difference it will make, there is a political consensus for action. The guiding principles of welfare and health reforms likely will not change radically, but the crisis has raised spending and state intervention to new levels and made them more legitimate. On the ground, despite the dire situation, unions had to threaten to strike in January 2021 to reach an agreement with private employers on wage hikes and to improve contracts in the elderly care sector where at least one in five still work by the hour.

In the Nordic region, Sweden is the country that has proven most open to new public management and privatization of welfare services (Blix and Jordahl, 2021). Most parties from Right to Left have endorsed these policies, which have deeply reshaped welfare and care. The official goals of these reforms were to improve freedom of choice and cost-efficiency of public investments through reducing bureaucracy and enhancing competition between providers. Politicians and researchers alike have debated these evolutions constantly over the last three decades, trying to appraise their impact on the nature of the Swedish model. The underlying ideological premise may well be that private – or mixed – solutions have to be developed for the provision of welfare services, and the risk is the production of a situation in which the more well-off decline to pay both for taxes that finance collective welfare and for top-ups to secure access to better services or insurance for their own sake. Although out-of-pocket expenses also have increased in Sweden, it seems that attachment to universal solutions and acquiescence to the relatively high taxes necessary to guarantee them remain comparatively high, even as voters have come to support right-wing parties (Svallfors, 2011; Blomqvist and Palme, 2020).

As a revealing epilogue in the political career of the government led by Stefan Löfven, a historic motion of no confidence was voted by parliament in June 2021. This was possible because the Left party doubted the government's intention to stop rent deregulation on the negotiated housing market. This issue was one of the most sensitive in the political pact that tied the Red–Green government to a 73-point liberal programme negotiated with the Right and including weakened labour protection and partial privatization of state employment service. Löfven shrewdly managed to come back one more time through the back door, on a different platform, but he was shaken and later announced he would quit as prime minister and party leader as of November 2021, when the Social Democratic Party congress was to be summoned. So it seemed that traditional welfare issues reframed by COVID-19 were set to be an integral part of the 2022 electoral campaign, at least until the new international crisis triggered by the war in Ukraine came along. Whether they will trigger new political alignments is not yet clear. It hinges on the duration of the current crisis, its influence on party manifestoes and the readiness to keep cooperating across political lines. What is clear, on the other hand, is the historic growth of direct government economic support and social compensation proportionate to the sheer scale and speed of the shock (Moreira and Hick, 2021). The high mortality in care homes, exacerbated by the heated debates around the Swedish strategy in 2020, fully exposed some of the weak spots of the Swedish decentralized and increasingly fragmented model of welfare. It triggered a response mostly by way of strong public investment and income and skills improvements, but it remains to be seen whether the precarious employment situation of some of the largest professional groups in the country may be addressed in turn. Another issue will be better coordination and integration between health care and elderly care so that the specific needs of a growing population of old and sometimes dependent people are taken care of. Finally, one of the biggest challenges of a universal social and health care model will be how to keep reaching out broadly to foreign-born populations and their descendants when a nationalist party is actively promoting welfare chauvinism and making inroads into Swedish society (Greve, 2020). Among the many reasons that may explain why these populations were more severely hit by COVID-19 is the fact that they provide part of the workforce for home care and other services that should be better valued.

The political and moral economy of the pandemic

The Swedish model discourse has always been politically and even normatively loaded. Sweden, along with the other Nordic countries, has come to epitomize evolving ideals of social and political progress, a different but successful world of welfare capitalism, to paraphrase Danish sociologist Gøsta Esping-Andersen. The pandemic crisis has brought about important changes that may have an impact on this image but also on a unitary conception of the Nordic model. Furthermore, it is questioning the nature and degree of trust within Swedish society that is usually regarded as a crucial component of the social fabric and one that played a role in supporting the specific approach in the pandemic.

The political uses of Sweden

The Nordic responses diverged in this crisis, maybe not so much in their intentions but at least on the level of discourses, policies and key actors. These divergences also triggered disagreements and sometimes tensions between decision makers but also between populations. Denmark, Finland and Norway were pictured as more reasonable, prudent and, perhaps, humane. Sweden has been in the spotlight, but not as usual for being one of the best in class. This time around, Sweden attracted a great deal of harsh criticism, especially from the political families that normally support one version or another of the Swedish model. Conversely, the Swedish line in the crisis has gained new supporters abroad who are not usually fans of social democratic politics, old or new. From libertarians to neoconservatives and all the way to different strands of national populists, many have looked to Sweden as a viable alternative to self-imposed general lockdowns of society. They suddenly praised the respect of civil liberties and sense of collective responsibility, the fact that businesses remained open, that a kind of social life was allowed to take place in bars and restaurants and, most importantly, that a political authority was not dictating to people how to behave but trusted them to do the right thing. Paradoxically, these unexpected supporters disregarded the fact that the Swedish welfare state played a significant role in buffering the effects of the crisis with its high and generous insurance coverage, free health care access, and exceptional compensation schemes specially tailored to the situation. High trust in these (welfare) state institutions and acquiescence to relatively high income taxes to finance them are also salient characteristics that do not sit well with the libertarian or neoconservative type of philosophy (Nguyen, 2020). In Sweden, in contrast, with a Social Democratic and Green alliance in power, critics mostly came from the Right, and even the nationalist party, which seemed self-defeating to progressives who witnessed the damage to the image of Swedish moral superiority (Palm, 2020).

Picturing Swedish policy as downright libertarian was certainly simplistic, and we have seen ample evidence now that alternatives were not between strict lockdown and some kind of hands-off herd immunity approach, as there were many shades of mitigation in between and many ways for local populations to adjust their behaviours. Since 2020 we have witnessed an impressive surge of contributions in media, academic publications and political discourses about the Swedish strategy. Many of them were searching for answers and points of comparison in times of uncertainty. As Fraser Nelson, editor of *The Spectator*, has it: Sweden was seen either as a 'liberal heaven or a Covid hell' (Nelson, 2020), but comparisons and analyses were often quite crude. We were flooded daily with statistics on infections, tests and death. There was a constant battle of figures to show that countries were performing better or worse, with indicators that had an extremely short-term bias and were often unweighted or not put in context. In other words, everyone could extract figures from various databases, sometimes for just a single day, and run comparisons on that basis to see which country had the highest number of cases or deaths.

More refined and sophisticated analyses have started to appear over time, giving a more complex evaluation of a Swedish case apparently riddled with high mortality. The data on excess mortality from one winter season allowed comparisons with previous years and a better assessment of the impact of COVID-19.[3] In a publication in the *British Medical Journal* studying 29 OECD countries, only three lacked excess mortality in 2020 as compared to a 2016–2019 baseline, namely Denmark, Norway and New Zealand. So, these countries were the exceptions, and two of them happened to be direct neighbours of Sweden.[4] The Swedish public authorities resorted to such statistics to show that their situation was not the anomaly it had been said to be, although it so happened that the other three Nordic countries fared exceptionally well in this pandemic. In this context, it should be remembered that only ten days prior to changing course drastically on 12 March, Norway also adopted a liberal approach, keeping it borders open even for travellers from Italy and insisting that 'the world must not stop' (Gjerde, 2020, p 263). Some senior Norwegian health experts also advised against school closure (at least at elementary levels) and did not recommend wearing masks at all times. In a June 2020 interview, the Norwegian director of public health, Camilla Stoltenberg, acknowledged that the differences between Scandinavian policies were probably less striking than had been depicted and that the effectiveness of specific measures was difficult to ascertain when countries had been exposed to different initial rates of infection (Unherd, 2020). The similarity of results is also reflected in the fact that Swedes 'voluntarily' reduced their daily movements in public spaces on a par with their Nordic neighbours, simply on the basis of recommendations to limit contacts.

Trust, consensus and conflicts

Sweden did not exactly epitomize a simple trade-off between liberty and security during this pandemic. Trust in public institutions and government is a key element and a shared value among the Nordic countries (Kumlin and Haugsgjerd, 2017). In times of national crisis, the legitimacy of public authorities may initially experience a boost due to a 'rally around the flag' effect (Andersson and Aylott, 2020). While many in Sweden and beyond were critical of what was perceived as a lack of direct government intervention, it is worth noting that the approval rates of the government and the prime minister went up decidedly at the start of the crisis, by some 20 points, from

45 to 65% and 25 to 45%, respectively. They subsequently declined to around 45 and 35% throughout 2020. This pattern is not specific to Sweden, as we can see almost the same trend for Boris Johnson and the British government, for instance. By comparison, trust in the Public Health Agency and Anders Tegnell followed roughly the same dynamic, but stayed above 60% at least until the end of 2020. The levels of trust in institutions and decision makers declined sharply during the first part of 2021 to reach historic lows (around 35% for Löfven, 50% for Tegnell and FHM). Yet general trust in government in 2020 went up decidedly from under 40% in 2019 to 65% in 2020 (Andersson and Oscarsson, 2020). This idea of trust has been mobilized time and again during the crisis as one of the main ingredients that can explain the Swedish resilience.

As Figure 2 shows, the level of trust in government is generally high and even higher when it comes to public administration. It is quite interesting to recall, as French sociologist Alain Gras did in a May 2020 op-ed, that Swedish crisis management strategies relied to a certain extent explicitly on this notion of trust. Gras referred to a Swedish public report from 2018 entitled 'to govern and lead with trust' in which we can find this citation of interesting comparative value by historian Lars Trägårdh, himself an active commentator during the COVID-19 crisis: 'In a society where bureaucrats and politicians lack trust in citizens, where democracy is weak or insignificant, or where the political culture is characterized by reciprocal distrust between citizens and authorities, the need for surveillance, control and repression is greater' (Trägårdh, 2018, p 407). Alain Gras emphasized the contrast with other governments, such as the French, that required citizens to follow the rules and act responsibly but at the same time changed the rules often and enforced a high number of controls (Gras, 2020). But I believe he overinterpreted the content of the study that aimed first and foremost at trust within public institutions and not between institutions and citizens (or the third dimension of interpersonal trust), although a correlation

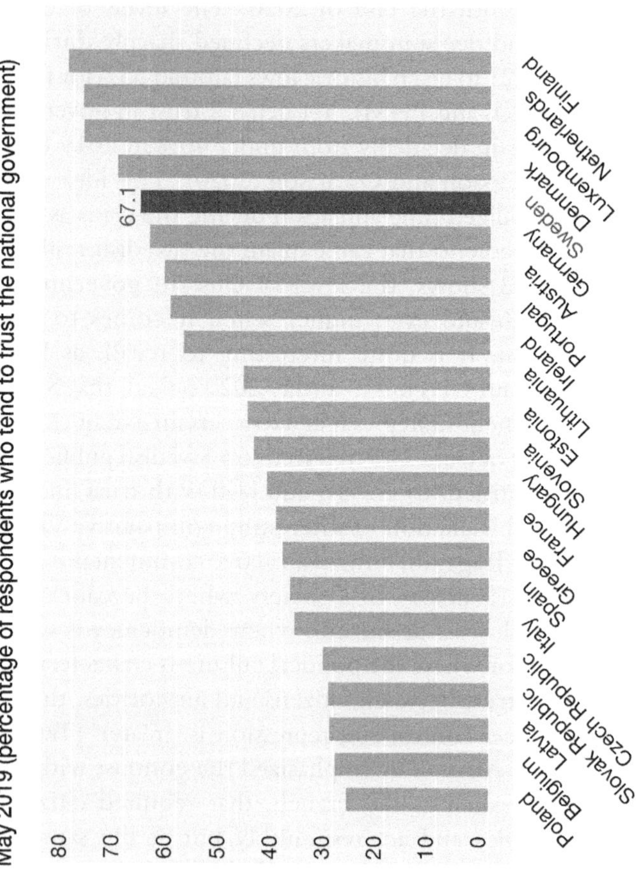

Figure 2: Average trust in the national government across the EU from November 2013 to May 2019 (percentage of respondents who tend to trust the national government)

Source: Data from https://data.oecd.org/gga/trust-in-government.htm

between these different dimensions certainly exists in Sweden. In any case, these different forms of trust were emphasized in the Swedish approach and were supposed to support its legitimacy. However, they were also put under heavy pressure because so much eventually depended on the judgement and recommendations of a few experts in a context of high scientific uncertainty and serious risks to human life. As Figure 2 shows, countries such as Denmark, Finland or even Germany exhibit a high level of trust in government as well but nevertheless chose a different approach. Yet, as Trägårdh and Özkirimli assume, 'in Sweden, the path chosen may be less draconian but it is possibly more demanding, since it shifts the burden from laws and policing to self-regulation' (Trägårdh and Özkirimli, 2020). It could be added that this self-regulation became the subject of intense scrutiny and judgement from a world in lockdown that tried to make some sense of the 'Swedish experiment' and, through this lens, of their own.

The pandemic has indeed polarized a Swedish society that tends to avoid conflicts, and it also triggered tensions with Nordic neighbours, particularly Norway. Facing outstanding criticism from abroad, part of the population stepped up in defence of a strategy perceived to be in line with Swedish values and culture. Yet all through the crisis discussions went on about the real independence of Swedish media that are partly financed by tax money and about the possibility of expressing critical opinions that would not be interpreted as national treason. This lack of independence was portrayed as the dark side of a consensus culture imposed from the top and contrasted with freedom of speech and a culture of openness (Lindström, 2020). A number of scientists and journalists have nevertheless gone public with open criticism of the Swedish strategy, and this occurred relatively early, as we have seen, in March and April 2020. Because Sweden stood alone and already faced quite a lot of foreign criticism for its handling of the pandemic, they were often accused of howling with the wolves or – perhaps more fittingly in this context – shooting at the ambulance (Jakobsen and Amundsen, 2021). As Andersson and Aylott argued, it was also plainly understandable from a pragmatic point of view that many people sided with policies that kept primary schools and day care open and maintained some essential social venues, such as bars and restaurants, in times when most other countries seemed to have closed them (Andersson and Aylott, 2020, p 232). On the other hand, even if COVID-19 raised the level of anxiety, we should be surprised by the results of serious opinion surveys that ranked the pandemic as only ninth among causes of anxiety for Swedes in 2020, behind crime, terrorism and climate change.[5]

It is perhaps not that Swedish people did not perceive the virus as a serious public health threat: they apparently did so on a par with Norwegians, according to early surveys, but the gradual response and pragmatic communication adopted by the authorities, added to the fact that life as usual did not stop at once in March, probably helped Swedes rationalize this epidemic differently, to such an extent that they could appear – from a distance – to be more impervious to the mounting death toll, particularly among the elderly.

Democracy, emergency and expert rule

Responses to the pandemic have mobilized exceptional powers and procedures in many countries, with states of emergency and special legislation, but the practice and potential abuse of these newly acquired powers have varied greatly (Greene 2020). In Hungary, crises have long been used as an excuse for reinforcing the executive's prerogatives under Viktor Orbán, leading to the so-called 'enabling act' of 23 March 2020 that gives the government almost full power. In France, the constitutional council judged that the 23 March organic law, installing a new regime of health emergency without the legally required 15-day delay before the vote, was legitimized by extraordinary circumstances, thus making possible the suspension of constitutional order in such cases. The state and constitutional councils were also completely absorbed by issues related to the pandemic, setting aside other pressing matters (Jacquin, 2020). On the other hand, New Zealand enforced a strict lockdown in the hope of eradicating COVID-19, but trod carefully from a legal standpoint, resorting to a state of emergency from 25 March to 13 May 2020 with seven-day reviews. The lockdown itself relied mostly on public health legislation and the appeals of Prime Minister Jacinda Ardern to the responsibility of all people (Knight, 2021).

In times of life-threatening crises, governments are likely to be judged on the efficacy of their response in spite of their consequences for the exercise of freedoms and rights. Some democratic regimes have gone quite far, overseeing contact tracing and quarantines through digital and phone tracking, dedicating important resources to the task. Such stringent policies were hailed as effective in South Korea and Taiwan whereas Western democracies were more reluctant to choose this path. But penalties for breach of confinement or quarantine have been severe even in the latter countries, with high fines (up to thousands of British pounds) and potential jail sentences. In several European countries, vaccine passports have also been introduced that create different categories of populations, severely restricting access to bars, restaurants and many public venues. At the very end of 2021, strangely even Sweden implemented such a passport but only for indoor gatherings exceeding 100 persons (later 50), triggering protests and demonstrations. The prolongation of the pandemic has raised important questions as to the duration and limitation of emergency orders or special powers that had already been used in recent times in relation to terrorist risks. Indeed, the elevated health risk could prove to be an existential threat to democracy, basic rights and freedom (Hennette-Vauchez, 2022). In the name of protecting populations against infection, public gatherings and demonstrations were banned or heavily controlled, elections could be postponed, parliaments were more likely to be sidelined, basic freedom of movement was severely restricted and health passports were implemented not only for travel but also for participation in daily activities. On the other hand, as we have seen, the pandemic led to a remarkable return to grace of the welfare state and public spending in a number of countries, although there may be a backlash in the longer run. This conjunction of restrictions and compensations – or protection – has been the subject of intense controversies (for example, regarding the biopolitical consequences of the crisis), reinforced by the climate of post-truth and conspiracy theories (Stiegler, 2020). Although legal challenges, debates and demonstrations have not stopped altogether, their legitimacy has been regularly opposed to a new imperative of safeguarding against one paramount health risk. Dissenters and protesters have run the risk of being cast as irresponsible and even criminal. The arrival of vaccines only confirmed this tendency, more or less simplistically reducing the alternatives to pro and con.

In this context, the case of Sweden strangely stands apart. Until recently, the country mostly followed the standard division of power, abided by constitutional and parliamentary procedures, respected the principle that grants responsibility to the same institutions in normal or crisis times and paid special attention to undue limitations of basic freedoms and rights. Nevertheless, decisions were made that gradually enforced more restrictions. A temporary pandemic legislation was finally implemented ten months after the start of the crisis, public inquiries on responsibilities were diligently carried out and broad consultations of organized social and political groups were maintained to secure consensus. However, the timing and necessities of democracy and crisis response may not coincide; if some governments possibly overreacted for fear of a catastrophe or sometimes because they could seize the opportunity to reinforce their power, as in Hungary, others may have underreacted, like the US under the Trump administration and, arguably, Sweden. In the Swedish case, the lack of certain legal instruments – such as provisions for a state of emergency – could be a hindrance in the short run, but, as we have seen in the span of 18 months, it was still possible to make stricter recommendations and implement more stringent restrictions on the basis of the constitution and the existing body of laws or to devise new statutes with a sunset clause (Baldwin, 2021, p 63). This is what Sweden ultimately did, extending its pandemic legislation and using it to implement a vaccine pass for larger events in December 2021. The scientific evaluation and forecast of the gravity of the crisis by official experts, the relative lack of material supplies and the fragmented system of health and crisis governance were also key elements in the difficult equation that each country tried to solve in its own sovereign way, with little international cooperation. Yet if initial conditions and mistakes are understood to account for the higher death rate compared to the other Nordic nations, they are not sufficient to explain why Sweden persisted so long in its specific response throughout the subsequent waves. There were some important adjustments at the end of 2020 but also strong elements of continuity all the way into the vaccination campaign in 2021.

Domestic actors often pictured this response as embedded in the specificities of a Swedish model of democratic and welfare governance, whereby the central government is but one component that does not have resources to act alone. Yet it is clear that this model reached some of its limits in the COVID-19 crisis and this is one of the main conclusions of the final report of the corona commission that advised to substantially beef up the expertise and coordination capacity of the government (Coronakommission, 2022). In other circumstances, Sweden has not always been such a keen defender of civil rights and liberties. It was not so liberal in the fight against previous epidemics and was much more regulationist with respect to AIDS, for instance. There were some problematic precedents, including a famous one that led to jurisprudence from the European Court of Human Rights in the case of *Enhorn v Sweden* in 2005. In this particular case, the court ruled that compulsory isolation of an HIV-positive man for 18 months in aggregate over a period of seven years to prevent him from spreading the virus was not legitimate and violated article 5.1 of the European Convention on Human Rights on 'the right to liberty and security'.[6]

Although the role of scientific expertise in politics and bureaucracy has been a central component of the Swedish – and Nordic – welfare regimes (Lundqvist and Petersen, 2010), the tendency has favoured a lesser role for experts, but the way it played out in Sweden during this crisis was clearly abnormal in this respect. While some heads of state or government went to the front lines in the battle against the virus, in Sweden it was a state epidemiologist and his public health agency that seemed to take the wheel and manage a good deal of the crisis communication. To be sure, this concentration on one man was in part an artefact of the encounter between the virus, scientific expertise and global media, yet it meant that this particular expert and his bureaucratic structure not only assumed a political and diplomatic role well beyond their normal functions but also epitomized a problematic form of (health) nationalism. Trying to make sense of this situation, Fabrizio Tassinari argued that 'it is less about voluntarism, responsibility and no lockdowns than about the government, its bureaucracy and its chief epidemiologist deciding how to protect people from themselves' (Tassinari, 2020). According to this view, behind the proclamations of equality, freedom and transparency lies the technocratic power of elites who can 'engineer painstaking consensus' and who rely on the high level of trust in society to do so. The deeply grounded reputation of Sweden as a fundamentally well-governed and moral democracy usually helps to obscure problems and avert criticism, but this time around the reserves of moral credit have been stretched thin. There are certainly good sides to a crisis communication that aims to defuse panic and social anxiety, unlike that in many other countries. This is also part of a Swedish educational programme that starts early in life and trains individuals to be wary of their information sources, to be alert to fake news and to trust official providers. But here again, the almost daily doses of Anders Tegnell's phlegmatic demeanour at press conferences for months on end took on an almost messianic dimension.

Yet, however central he appeared to be through the mediatic lens, the Swedish state epidemiologist was not the only architect behind choices, recommendations and decisions. All levels of society and politics were mobilized, from individuals to businesses, media and political parties. Collective choices had to be made and justified, and risks and benefits had to be assessed not only in the short term but also on a longer timescale, the most immediate and brutal cost being the tragic loss of human lives. In comparison, not much was made in foreign media of the 18 million farmed minks Denmark culled and hastily buried in a matter of days in fear of a possible virus mutation in November 2020, although it led to a domestic political crisis called the 'minkgate' and to a special commission of inquiry (Bergkvist, 2021). In locked-down countries or in Sweden, the same people were more likely to be exposed and vulnerable to the virus: the elderly in need of assistance, people working in 'essential services' (whether health care or supermarkets) and also all those who could not so easily isolate themselves because of their housing, economic and health conditions (Suhonen, 2020). Evaluation of the larger costs and consequences of this pandemic at different levels will continue, as the story is far from being over and the virus seems to be here to stay in one form or another. As time goes by, the exceptionality of the Swedish response will most likely fade away, but for now the impact on this democratic and welfare society and on its image should not be underestimated, leaving open questions as to the political and institutional changes that are desirable.

Conclusion

On 29 September 2021, Sweden was among the first countries –
with Denmark and Norway – to lift all the restrictions related
to COVID-19. Between 65 and 75% of the residents of the
Nordic countries were fully vaccinated at the time, but the
rollout was considered strong enough. In Sweden, the special
pandemic legislation remained in place until the beginning
of 2022. After a year and a half, the Nordic region returned
to some sense of normalcy, and Sweden was no longer the
outlier or the quasi-pariah state that it had been. The situation
in Sweden posed a striking contrast to that of countries like
Russia, which in autumn 2021 were seeing new peaks in
infections and death rates along with low vaccination levels.

Nevertheless, Figure 3 reminds us of the markedly
different impact of COVID-19 as measured by fatalities
directly associated with the virus among the countries of
northern Europe.

In proportion to the population, the Swedish death rate
is at about 1,450 deaths per million people, which was
significantly lower than the French (1,730), the British
(2,020), the Italian (2,150) or the Belgian (2,200) rate but
still much higher than rates of neighbouring nations. The
measure of excess mortality (that is, death from all causes in
a given year as compared to what should be expected from
data for several previous years) is commonly believed to give
a more accurate estimate of the true impact of COVID-19,
provided that demographic statistics can be trusted. Seen in
this light, and although calculation methods can vary,[1] excess
mortality in Sweden was high during four or five months of
2020, with peaks in April and December and very high for
the age category over 75, but the average deviation was still

Figure 3: COVID-19-related fatalities in the Nordic countries, as of September 2021

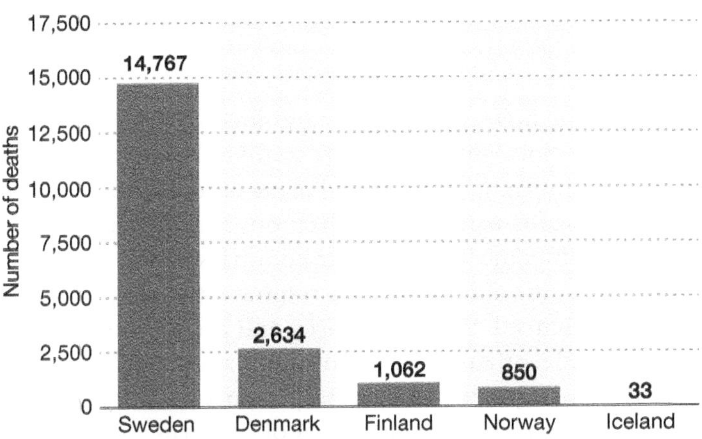

Source: Statista, Nordics: coronavirus deaths 2022, Statista

among the lowest in Europe. According to Eurostat, Swedish excess mortality increased by 6.5% in 2020 as compared to the baseline of 2016–2019, with corresponding figures of 12% for France, 18% for Belgium and up to 20% for Spain, while Denmark stood at 2%. The European average was nearly 12% higher than the baseline.[2]

As important as the death count may be, the absolute and relative impact of a pandemic like this one (which is not finished) goes well beyond mortality caused by the new virus and will take more time to assess (Gaudillière et al., 2021). Richard Horton, the editor of the scientific journal *The Lancet*, referred to the concept of 'syndemic' to address the COVID-19 impact's extreme diversity, not only between nations, but also within them:

> The total number of people living with chronic diseases is growing. Addressing COVID-19 means addressing hypertension, obesity, diabetes, cardiovascular and chronic respiratory diseases, and cancer. Paying greater

> attention to NCDs [noncommunicable diseases] is not an agenda only for richer nations. NCDs are a neglected cause of ill-health in poorer countries too. (Horton, 2020)

In this sense, how governments and media reacted did and will matter a lot. For instance, the warlike rhetoric of French President Emmanuel Macron and many other political leaders set the tone for national mobilizations that did not reflect the sharp differences across their countries in the ways that both the virus and the public response to the pandemic were experienced. Some territories and age categories were spared, while others suffered disproportionately. In other cases, as in Brazil, a parliamentary report recently showed that President Bolsonaro's dismissal of the virus and vaccines should be viewed as a crime against humanity. As of October 2021, Brazil had the second-most absolute deaths after the US, over 600,000, and the report holds that at least 100,000 could have been avoided, particularly among the indigenous populations. In Sweden, although there was also a form of national mobilization to mitigate the spread, the pandemic response was more gradual, and authorities were more reluctant to resort to drastic measures that were difficult to implement from a legal and constitutional point of view. This response appeared to be in line with the normal division of work among government, agencies and local authorities as well as with the existing pandemic emergency plans. It was mostly based on recommendations, delivered with a communication style meant to deter panic and to induce cooperation of the population, in anticipation that the virus would stay. However, it could also be regarded as a blatant underestimation of some of the risks incurred with COVID-19 (Claeson and Hanson, 2020). It underscored the failing coordination between the multiple layers of autonomous institutions and raised questions about the political capacity to steer the country in such a crisis. The contrast with a majority of countries as to going into more or less strict and durable lockdown of the entire population in spring 2020 triggered considerable attention to what was increasingly regarded as a 'Swedish experiment', although it was arguably no less of an experiment than the total confinement of a society. Indeed, many countries entered uncharted territory during these uncertain times, enacting exceptional measures and legislation that substantially affected freedoms and rights as well as socioeconomic activities.

The deviant Swedish response, I have argued in this book, is both coherent with a certain number of institutional specificities and paradoxical in many ways. It can be accounted for by a conjunction of factors, without disregarding political and personal dimensions such as the weakness of governments since 2014 and the particular profile of the prime minister, Stefan Löfven, and of the state epidemiologist, Anders Tegnell. If Swedish public agencies traditionally enjoy strong autonomy in relation to government and individual ministries, they hardly ever reach the degree of predominance and visibility achieved by FHM and by one single expert. Anders Tegnell and some of his colleagues came to play a highly political and diplomatic role in defence of decisions to shun the two most salient and new policies of lockdown and mask mandates until vaccination came about. Strangely enough, the Swedish authorities eventually decided on a vaccine pass when its immunization level was already high. Crisis management also raised questions, because Sweden had pandemic plans and a reasonable degree of preparation derived from earlier experiences, but the decentralized, fragmented and overloaded health and social care services made it hard to implement coherent, timely and efficient measures across the country on the basis of simple public health 'recommendations'.

All along there was a specific framing of this distinct approach in foreign and domestic media that resorted to the classic trope of Swedish exceptionality, but the values of progressiveness that are usually associated with that trope were put under severe strain, and the patterns of political support of the Swedish model abroad were notably transformed this time around. An unexpected coalition of neoconservatives, libertarians and national-populists outside Sweden came to pay tribute to the Swedish defence of freedoms, civil rights and small businesses, while Swedish authorities had to deploy diplomatic efforts to convince many sceptical governments that they were not acting recklessly. In doing so, they also insisted that their approach was coherent with their institutions, with values of social trust, with respect for the rule of law and ultimately with the goal to mitigate the overall effects of the pandemic. Conflicting political uses of the Swedish reference may have intensified in recent years with the development of global social media in an era of post-truth, yet they are not really such a new phenomenon. They have certainly contributed to the ambivalence and conceptual flexibility of the idea of a progressive Swedish model that also proved to be the instrument of an exceptional nation-branding strategy. It is even possible that this deeply problematic visibility that Sweden gained during the pandemic can be converted into something positive now that Sweden is back on the more familiar terrain of global solidarity to distribute vaccines more equally across the world.

The controversies surrounding the Swedish approach to the pandemic have revolved around the buzzword of herd immunity – in the sense of immunity acquired through infections – and the possibility that experts were performing some kind of natural experiment on the population, with deadly consequences. There is no denying that a degree of such immunity was hoped for as a side-effect from a virus that spread quickly in spring 2020, but if this was the main guiding principle, there was a contradiction in recommendations to work from home, limit contacts and employ remote learning for all levels but primary schools. After it became clear that levels of immunity were lower than expected, the Swedish options did not change radically, although restrictions were tightened and new pandemic legislation formally gave more leeway to the government eight months after the start of the crisis.

The scientific consensus on the coronavirus may have taken time to solidify, yet Sweden tended to steer away from it and even from certain WHO recommendations, as evidenced by the very late and gradual change of doctrine on the selective use of masks or on the airborne nature of the virus. It is quite clear, in this respect, that scientific and statistical data have been used and twisted in all sorts of ways during this crisis, especially in the service of 'health nationalism' and competition, both of which reached startling proportions. Sweden was not at all immune to these tendencies, and part of the population responded to the climate of Sweden-bashing by showing relatively strong support to the people in charge of the crisis response, most notably Anders Tegnell, who was arguably one of the only chief epidemiologists to attract so many antagonistic passions – standing between the extremes of national hero and criminal.

Swedish society came out more deeply divided, especially between those who believed that the response had been proportionate to the risks, in line with Swedish values and respectful of the capacity of people to act responsibly and those who considered that the price paid in mortality – particularly among the very old and frail and the migrant populations living in urban neighbourhoods – was way too high and could have been reduced through earlier and slightly more stringent measures. The Swedish media have been accused of being far too uncritical and of channelling views along a narrow 'opinion corridor'. In any case, the Swedish strategy received a fair amount of criticism from foreign media, and the Swedish media were certainly not simply releasing the holy words of Anders Tegnell. Beyond the watchdog function of the mediasphere, Sweden was one of the first countries to set up a public commission of inquiry, which issued its first, preliminary report within six months in 2020, severely faulting the fragmented and slow response and its role in the high mortality rate in care homes during the first wave. The next reports in 2021–22 emphasised the disproportionate impact of early decisions based on available evidence rather than on a more precautionary principle in the face of a new virus. They by and large supported the liberal approach that limited the weight of undue restrictions and they lauded the role of the government not only to compensate for hardships but also to support economic recovery. However, the commission made it clear that some of the instruments acquired by the government only in 2021 could and should have been developed earlier on to improve national coordination and raise the level of political leadership (Coronakommissionen, 2020; 2021; 2022). Swedish decision makers eventually started to come to terms with some of the failings of the epidemic response, though they did not so radically change course, suggesting that their specific mitigation policy was still legitimate.

In many ways, however, COVID-19 has placed the Swedish model under unprecedented cross-pressures, affecting some of the sensitive areas of welfare, social and health care that have been subject to continuous reforms and debates and are considered to be key points in the neoliberal mutation of the Swedish welfare system: health and hospital care, elderly care, unemployment insurance and compensation. To a large extent, health and care institutions and policies are decentralized in Sweden and have been a terrain for many reforms inspired by new public management and marketization programmes that added new layers of complexity to existing structural problems. Because of all the havoc that it wreaked, the pandemic has triggered some renewal of debates on these matters as well as initiatives to improve the situation, especially for elderly care, and as the country is moving into an election year in 2022. It should be added that immigrants and the policies directed to this category of population, another central and divisive political issue in recent years, have featured prominently in the pandemic crisis. Indeed, if the virus was most likely brought into Sweden courtesy of well-off tourists returning from the Alpine ski resorts, the first major clusters were found in much less well-off suburban areas of Stockholm where old and new migrant populations have flocked. Some of these minority groups and urban areas have been more impacted by COVID-19 and its adverse socioeconomic consequences, reminding of the real weight of these structural inequalities.

In these extraordinary times characterized by increased state intervention, central political command, national retrenchment, mobilization and emergency orders, the Swedish approach could carry appeal as a more liberal and pragmatic alternative to mitigate the overall effects of the pandemic while learning to live with this new virus. The Swedes did not expect either that their neighbours and many other welfare states would make radically different choices or that vaccines would arrive so soon. Yet they hung on steadfastly to the line they had taken as a reflection of a typical Swedish order likely to secure popular support, although it increasingly deviated into a form of health nationalism. The relatively high mortality, especially among the elderly, nevertheless cast a shadow on the image of a progressive Swedish model and deeply split the 'people's home'.[3] There will be hard lessons to learn from this crisis in order to demonstrate the resilience of Swedish democracy and welfare in the future, yet few societies will be spared this daunting challenge of self-examination.

Notes

Chapter 1

[1] www.aftonbladet.se/nyheter/a/zg0dwq/jo-avvisar-forslag-till-pandemilag

[2] At a 2017 rally, Trump referred to Sweden as if something really serious had happened, such as a terrorist attack, but nothing of the kind had occurred.

[3] The literature in this area is massive. For a general and comparative analysis, see Kananen (2016).

[4] https://data.oecd.org/pension/net-pension-replacement-rates.htm. Unemployment insurance replacement rates are on the rise again since 2010, but the share of the unemployed eligible for earnings-related benefits has been halved in 15 years (Nelson, 2017, p 290).

[5] www.scb.se/en/finding-statistics/statistics-by-subject-area/labour-market/labour-force-surveys/labour-force-surveys-lfs/pong/statistical-news/labour-force-surveys-lfs-annual-averages-2020/

Chapter 2

[1] https://data.oecd.org/healtheqt/hospital-beds.htm

[2] However, some venues, such as schools or libraries, were not directly concerned, and there was no regulation on private gatherings other than voluntary ones.

[3] *Pressträff* [COVID-19 daily Press conference], 17 March 2020, my translation.

[4] www.rnz.co.nz/national/programmes/sunday/audio/2018746794/johan-giesecke-why-lockdowns-are-the-wrong-approach

[5] www.riksrevisionen.se/rapporter/granskningsrapporter/2008/pandemier---hantering-av-hot-mot-manniskors-halsa.html

[6] www.dinsakerhet.se/siteassets/dinsakerhet.se/broschyren-om-krisen-eller-kriget-kommer/om-krisen-eller-kriget-kommer---engelska-2.pdf

[7] www.icfj.org/news/swedens-top-epidemiologist-challenges-conventional-wisdom-covid-19

[8] This is my translation from the original Swedish: www.folkhalsomyndigheten.se/contentassets/b6cce03c4d0e4e7ca3c9841bd96e6b3a/pandemiberedskap-hur-vi-forbereder-oss-19074-1.pdf

[9] Ulf Kristersson, *Statsministerns frågestund* [Questions to the prime minister], 17 March, my translation.

10 Stefan Löfven, official speech to the nation, 22 March 2020, my translation.

11 *Sverige och tsunamin – granskning och förslag* (SOU 2005:104).

12 *Utredningen om hälso- och sjukvårdens beredskap* (S2018:09).

13 The amendment (Prop. 2019/20:155) concerned mostly public gatherings, shopping malls, social and cultural activities and transportation.

Chapter 3

1 What I intended to express was that the Swedish response may appear as a search for collective immunity that did not say its name, in spite of public recommendations to be very cautious.

2 https://sverigesradio.se/artikel/7473277

3 https://elcomercio.pe/mundo/europa/coronavirus-la-arriesgada-apuesta-de-suecia-de-luchar-contra-el-covid-19-protegiendo-la-economia-y-la-libertad-ciudadana-noticia/, my translation.

4 www.wort.lu/de/international/schwedens-corona-sonderweg-mit-hohem-preis-5e9ead51da2cc1784e35c146

5 See Kettunen and Petersen (2022) for a good overview of this blossoming literature.

6 www.regeringen.se/regeringens-politik/regeringens-arbete-med-coronapandemin/strategi-med-anledning-av-det-nya-coronaviruset

7 www.youtube.com/watch?v=WMPxwWa4F9o&list=PLw2eBi2rSx3bo5OxqM8y6qbecq7_MwOlt&index=230

8 www.tv4play.se/program/nyhetsmorgon/folkh%C3%A4lsomyndigheten-om-coronaviruset-man-ska-f%C3%B6rbereda-sig/12528736

9 www.un.org/fr/coronavirus/articles/recommandations-port-du-masque

10 www.who.int/director-general/speeches/detail/who-director-general-s-opening-remarks-at-the-media-briefing-on-covid-19---5-june-2020

11 Pressträff (COVID-19 Press conference), 24 February 2020 (www.regeringen.se/pressmeddelanden/2020/02/presstraff-med-anledning-av-coronaviruset/).

12 www.who.int/docs/default-source/coronaviruse/transcripts/who-audio-emergencies-coronavirus-press-conference-29apr2020.pdf?sfvrsn=aaa81d24_2, p 12

13 It also resulted in the setting up of an alternative organization and website for information on the pandemic, Vetenskapsforum Covid-19 https://vetcov19.se/

14 Although it was legally impossible in the short term to lock down entirely, FHM could have advised complete school closure and quarantines for inbound travellers.

15 https://ambstoccolma.esteri.it/ambasciata_stoccolma/it/ambasciata/news/dall_ambasciata/2020/03/comunicato-stampa-dell-ambasciatore.html

16 www.facebook.com/groups/797526950758017/, my translation.

Chapter 4

1   https://tv.aftonbladet.se/video/312101/jimmie-aakesson-inte-bara-ett-misslyckande-det-ar-en-massaker

2   www.france24.com/fr/europe/20200911-anders-tegnell-%C3%A9pid%C3%A9miologiste-en-chef-de-la-su%C3%A8de-nous-sommes-satisfaits-de-notre-strat%C3%A9gie

3   www.post-gazette.com/opinion/2020/11/10/The-ongoing-Swedish-experiment-COVID-Sweden/stories/202010200072; www.eltiempo.com/politica/gobierno/la-estrategia-de-suecia-contra-el-coronavirus-que-colombia-estudia-548382

4   https://assets.publishing.service.gov.uk/government/uploads/system/uploads/attachment_data/file/931005/S0762_Fifty-seventh_SAGE_meeting_on_Covid-19.pdf

5   www.krisinformation.se/en/news/2020/november. The new restrictions were initially implemented for a period of four weeks.

6   Prime minister's speech, www.youtube.com/watch?v=NSjik8P-LKk.

7   Parliamentary questions to the prime minister, www.riksdagen.se/sv/webb-tv/video/statsministerns-fragestund/statsministerns-fragestund_H7C120200319sf; my translation.

8   Similarly, the national ban on nursing home visits hurriedly reintroduced in November 2020 was later tailored locally.

9   https://medicalxpress.com/news/2020-11-narcolepsy-fiasco-spurs-covid-vaccine.html

10 Covax is a facility backed by the GAVI and the WHO.

11 www.aninews.in/news/world/asia/swedish-pm-lofven-appreciates-indias-role-as-pharmacy-of-the-world20210305191323/

12 www.tribuneindia.com/news/nation/covid-19-sweden-working-closely-with-partners-in-india-says-envoy-252364

13 www.government.se/government-of-sweden/ministry-for-foreign-affairs/

14 https://unric.org/sv/covid-19-de-drabbas-mest-och-vaccineras-minst/

15 www.regeringen.se/artiklar/2020/12/regeringen-valkomnar-coronakommissionens-delbetankande/

16 There has been a debate over changing this job title and eliminating the prefix 'under'.

[17] Prime minister Olof Palme, shot in Stockholm in 1986, and Foreign Minister Anna Lindh, stabbed to death in a department store in 2003.

[18] However, a very critical report by MPs on the early COVID-19 response was published in October 2021. It did not prevent the Conservatives from staying atop opinion polls until stories of parties at Downing Street started to surface and triggered a new inquiry early in 2022.

Chapter 5

[1] www.regeringen.se/regeringens-politik/socialforsakringar/atgarder-inom-sjukforsakringen-med-anledning-av-corona/.

[2] In December 2020, another inquiry in relation to the pandemic context was started, and a report is expected in 2022 (www.sou.gov.se/aldreomsorg/).

[3] When reported COVID-19 deaths are much lower than excess mortality, one may infer that COVID-19 mortality has been underestimated.

[4] Finland and South Korea also evidenced minor excess mortality.

[5] www.gu.se/som-institutet/resultat-och-publikationer/som-underso kningen-om-coronaviruset

[6] http://hudoc.echr.coe.int/eng?i=001-68077

Conclusion

[1] In particular the baseline can be five years, four years or sometimes only the previous year. It can be an average of these years or a formula that accounts for the year-to-year change over the entire period.

[2] https://ec.europa.eu/eurostat/databrowser/view/demo_r_mwk_ts/default/table?lang=en

[3] This is the translation of *folkhemmet*, a highly popular expression to describe Swedish society and its intrinsic solidarity.

References

Ahlenius, I-B. (2020) 'Regeringen har abdikerat', *Kvartal*, [online], https://kvartal.se/artiklar/regeringen-har-abdikerat

Ahlström, K. et al (2020) 'Därför blev svenskarna folkhälsopatrioter', *Dagens Nyheter*, [online] 13 May, www.dn.se/kultur-noje/darfor-blev-svenskarna-folkhalsopatrioter/

Amnesty International (2020) *As if Expendable: The UK Government's Failure to Protect Older People in Care Homes during the COVID-19 Pandemic*, London, Peter Benenson House, [online], www.amnesty.org.uk/care-homes-report

Anderberg, J. (2021) *Flocken. Berättelsen om hur Sverige Valde Väg under Pandemin*, Stockholm, Albert Bonniers Förlag

Andersson, C. and Pryser Libell, H. (2020) 'Finland, "Prepper Nation of the Nordics," Isn't Worried About Masks', *The New York Times*, [online] 5 April, www.nytimes.com/2020/04/05/world/europe/coronavirus-finland-masks.html

Andersson, J. (2009a) 'Nordic Nostalgia and Nordic Light: The Swedish model as Utopia 1930–2007', *Scandinavian Journal of History*, 34(3), 229–245

Andersson, J. (2009b) *The Library and the Workshop. Social Democracy and Capitalism in the Knowledge Age*, Stanford, Stanford University Press

Andersson, S. and Aylott, N. (2020) 'Sweden and Coronavirus: Unexceptional Exceptionalism', *Social Sciences*, 9(12), 232–250, https://doi.org/10.3390/socsci9120232

Andersson, U. and Oscarsson, H. (2020) 'Institutionsförtroendet inte lika politiserat under pandemin', SOM-Institutet, Göteborgs Universitet [report], https://www.gu.se/sites/default/files/2020-10/4.%20Institutionsf%C3%B6rtroendet%20inte%20lika%20politiserat%20under%20pandemin.pdf

Aschwanden, C. (2021) 'Five Reasons Why COVID Herd Immunity is Probably Impossible', *Nature*, [online] 18 March, www.nature.com/articles/d41586-021-00728-2

Aucante, Y. (2013a) *Les Démocraties Scandinaves: Des Systèmes Politiques Exceptionnels?*, Paris, Armand Colin

Aucante, Y. (2013b) 'L'antimodèle: les racines de la critique de la social-démocratie en Suède après 1945', *Nordiques*, 25, 23–35

Aucante, Y. and Aucante, N. (2017) *Icelandic Revolutions*, [documentary film], www.ehess.fr/fr/media/icelandic-revolutions

Aucante, Y. (2020a) 'Paradoxes of Hegemony: Scandinavian Social Democracy and the State', in M. Fulla and M. Lazar (eds) *European Socialists and the State*, London, Palgrave McMillan, 97–119

Aucante, Y. (2020b) 'Covid-19: L'exception suédoise', *Libération.fr*, [online] 10 April, www.liberation.fr/debats/2020/04/10/covid-19-l-exception-suedoise_1784816/?redirected=1

Bäckström Johansson, M. (2021) 'Pandemilag bör inte användas för lockdown', *Svenska Dagbladet*, [online] 7 January, www.svd.se/pandemilag-bor-inte-anvandas-for-lockdown

Baekkeskov, E. and Rubin, O. (2014) 'Why Pandemic Response is Unique: Powerful Experts and Hands-Off Political Leaders', *Disaster Prevention and Management*, 23(1), 81–93, www.emerald.com/insight/content/doi/10.1108/DPM-05-2012-0060/full/html?skipTracking=true

Baldwin, P. (2021) *Fighting the First Wave: Why the Coronavirus Was Tackled So Differently Across the Globe*, Harvard, Cambridge University Press

Bandelow, N.C. et al (2021) 'Patterns of Democracy Matter in the COVID-19 Crisis A Comparison of French and German Policy Processes', *International Review of Public Policy*, 3(1), 1–18, https://doi.org/10.4000/irpp.1788

Bankel, A-K. et al (2020) 'Arbetsmiljöverkets inspektör avslöjar spelet om munskydden', *Svt Nyheter*, [online] 28 October, www.svt.se/nyheter/granskning/ug/arbetsmiljoverkets-inspektor-avslojar-spelet-om-munskydden-rattsvidriga-saker

Barker, V. (2018) *Nordic Nationalism and Penal Order: Walling the Welfare State*, London, Routledge

Batchelor, O. (2020) 'Brostrøm: Grænselukning er en ren politisk beslutning', *DR.DK*, [online] 14 March, www.dr.dk/nyheder/indland/brostroem-graenselukning-er-en-ren-politisk-beslutning

Becker, P. and Bynander, F. (2017) 'The System for Crisis Management in Sweden: Collaborative, Conformist, Contradictory', in C.N. Madu and C. Kuei (eds) *Handbook of Disaster Risk Reduction & Management*, Singapore, World Scientific, 69–95, https:// doi. org/10.1142/10392

Belfrage, C. and Kallifatides, M. (2018) 'Financialisation and the New Swedish Model', *Cambridge Journal of Economics*, 42(4), 875–900, https://doi.org/10.1093/cje/bex089

Bentzen, N. et al (2020) States of Emergency in Response to the Coronavirus Crisis: Situation in Certain Member States, Brussels, European Parliament [briefing], www.europarl. europa.eu/RegData/etudes/BRIE/2020/651972/EPRS_ BRI(2020)651972_EN.pdf

Bergeron, H. and Castel, P. (2018) *Sociologie Politique de la Santé* (2nd edn), Paris, PUF

Bergeron H. et al (2020) *Covid-19: Une Crise Organisationnelle*, Paris, Presses de Sciences Po

Berggren, J. and Martinsson, K. (2018) 'Tre undersköterskor: Så kan vår arbetsmiljö bli bättre', *Arbetet*, [online] 9 November, https://arbetet.se/2018/11/09/tre-underskoterskor-sa-kan-var-arbetsmiljo-bli-battre/

Bergh, A. (2013) 'What are the Policy Lessons from Sweden? On the Rise, Fall and Revival of a Capitalist Welfare State', *New Political Economy*, 19(5), 662–694, https://doi.org/10.1080/ 13563467.2013.849670

Bergkvist, F. (2021) 'Danmarks statsminister kan ställas inför riksrätt', *Dagens Nyheter*, [online] 7 October, www.dn.se/varlden/ danmarks-statsminister-kan-stallas-infor-riksratt/

Berglund, T. et al (2020) 'Occupational Change on the Dualised Swedish Labour Market', *Economic and Industrial Democracy*, October 2020, https://doi:10.1177/0143831X20959714

Bergman, A. (2007) 'Co-Constitution of Domestic and International Welfare Obligations: The Case of Sweden's Social Democratically Inspired Internationalism', *Cooperation and Conflict*, 42(1), 73–99, http://www.jstor.org/stable/45084439

Berlivet, L. and Löwy, I. (2020) 'Hydroxychloroquine Controversies: Clinical Trials, Epistemology, and the Democratization of Science', *Medical Anthropology Quarterly*, 34(4), 525–541, https://pubmed.ncbi.nlm.nih.gov/33210338/

Blanck, A. (2021) 'Fördelningen av vacciner måste bli mer rättvis', *Dagens Industri* [online] 19 May, www.di.se/debatt/fordelningen-av-vacciner-maste-bli-mer-rattvis/

Blix, M. and Jordahl, H. (2021) *Privatizing Welfare Services: Lessons from the Swedish Experiment*, Oxford, Oxford University Press

Blomqvist, P. and Palme, J. (2020) 'Universalism in Welfare Policy: The Swedish Case beyond 1990', *Social Inclusion*, 8(1), 114–123 https://doi:10.17645/si.v8i1.2511

Blomqvist, P. and Winblad, U. (2020) 'Contracting Out Welfare Services: How are Private Contractors Held Accountable?', *Public Management Review*, 27 September, https://doi.org/10.1080/14719037.2020.1817530

Blume, E. (2020) 'Björn Olsen: De bästa forskarna finns inte på Folkhälsomyndigheten', *Fokus*, [online] 20 March, www.fokus.se/2020/03/bjorn-olsen-coronaviruset-nar-sin-kulmen-i-sverige-om-nagra-veckor/

Booth, M. (2015) *The Almost Nearly Perfect People: Behind the Myth of the Scandinavian Utopia*, New York, Random House

Bricco, J. et al (2020) 'What are the Economic Effects of Pandemic Containment Policies? Evidence from Sweden', *IMF Working Paper* 20/191, [online], www.imf.org/en/Publications/WP/Issues/2020/09/18/What-are-the-Economic-Effects-of-Pandemic-Containment-Policies-Evidence-from-Sweden-49706

Broberg, G. and Roll-Hansen, N. (1996) *Eugenics and the Welfare State: Sterilization Policy in Denmark, Sweden, Norway, and Finland*, East Lansing, Michigan State University Press

Brommesson, D. (2018) 'Introduction to Special Section: From Nordic Exceptionalism to a Third Order Priority – Variations of "Nordicness" in Foreign and Security Policy', *Global Affairs* 4(4–5), 355–362, https://doi.org/10.1080/23340460.2018.1533385

Browning, C. (2007) 'Branding Nordicity: Models, Identity and the Decline of Exceptionalism', *Cooperation and Conflict*, 42(1), 27–51, https//doi:10.1177/0010836707073475

Busch, E. (2020) 'Våga tala klarspråk om corona och förorten', *Aftonbladet*, [online] 2 April, www.aftonbladet.se/debatt/a/naxyEm/vaga-tala-klarsprak-om-corona-och-fororten

Cameron, I. and Jonsson-Cornell, A. (2020) 'Sweden and COVID 19: A Constitutional Perspective', *Verfassungsblog*, [online] 7 May, https://verfassungsblog.de/sweden-and-covid-19-a-constitutional-perspective/

Capano, G. et al (2020) 'Mobilizing Policy (In)Capacity to Fight COVID-19: Understanding Variations in State Responses', *Policy and Society*, 39(3), 285–308, https://doi.org/10.1080/14494035.2020.1787628

Castles, F.G. (1978) *The Social Democratic Image of Society: A Study of the Achievements and Origins of Scandinavian Social Democracy in Comparative Perspective*, Boston, Routledge & Kegan

Castro, A. (2020) 'El caso (no tan) atípico de Suecia frente al Covid-19', *El Sol de México*, [online] 31 March, www.elsoldemexico.com.mx/mundo/suecia-control-coronavirus-caso-no-tan-atipico-covid-19-sin-cuarentena-5041023.html

Cauchemez, S. et al (2009) 'Closure of Schools During an Influenza Pandemic', *The Lancet*, 9(8), 473–481, https//doi: 10.1016/S1473-3099(09)70176-8

Cedervall Lauta, K. (2020) 'Something is Forgotten in the State of Denmark: Denmark's Response to the COVID-19 Pandemic', *Verfassungsblog*, [online] 4 May, https://verfassungsblog.de/something-is-forgotten-in-the-state-of-denmark-denmarks-response-to-the-covid-19-pandemic/

Chartier, D. (2011) *The End of Iceland's Innocence: The Image of Iceland in the Foreign Media during the Financial Crisis*, Ottawa, University of Ottawa Press

Childs, M.W. (1936) *Sweden: The Middle Way*, London, Faber & Faber

Childs, M.W. (1938) *This is Democracy: Collective Bargaining in Scandinavia*, New Haven, Yale University Press

REFERENCES

Christiansen, M. et al (2008) 'The Law of Communicable Diseases Act and Disclosure to Sexual Partners Among HIV-Positive Youth, *Vulnerable Child Youth Studies*, 3(3), 234–242, http://doi: 10.1080/17450120802069109

Claeson, M. and Hanson, S. (2020) 'COVID-19 and the Swedish Enigma', *The Lancet*, 397(10271), 259–261, https://doi.org/10.1016/S0140-6736(20)32750-1

Clark, R. (2020) 'Lockdown Supporters Cannot Bear the Thought that Sweden has Got it Right', *The Telegraph*, [online] 9 August, www.telegraph.co.uk/news/2020/08/09/lockdown-supporters-cannot-bear-thought-sweden-has-got-right

Clerc, L. et al (eds) (2015) *Histories of Public Diplomacy and Nation Branding in the Nordic and Baltic Countries: Representing the Periphery*, Leiden, Brill

Clerc, L. and Glover, N. (2015) 'Representing the Small States of Northern Europe: Between Imagined and Imaged Communities', in L. Clerc et al (eds) *Histories of Public Diplomacy and Nation Branding in the Nordic and Baltic Countries: Representing the Periphery*, Leiden, Brill, 1–20

Cohen, N. (2020) 'Welcome to Libertarian Covid Fantasy Land – that's Sweden to You and Me', *The Guardian*, [online] 26 September, www.theguardian.com/commentisfree/2020/sep/26/welcome-to-libertarian-covid-fantasy-land-thats-sweden-to-you-and-me

Collste, G. (2020) 'Ge förortens invånare förtur till vaccin', *Dagens Arena*, [online] 27 December, www.dagensarena.se/opinion/ge-forortens-invanare-fortur-till-vaccin/

Coronakommissionen (2020) Äldreomsorgen under pandemin. *Delbetänkande*, Stockholm, Statens Offentliga Utredningar, SOU 2020:80

Coronakommissionen (2021) *Sverige under pandemyn*, 2 volumes, Stockholm, Statens Offentliga Utredningar, SOU 2021:89

Coronakommissionen (2022) *Sverige under pandemyn*, 2 volumes, Stockholm, Statens Offentliga Utredningar, SOU 2022:10

Cox, R. (2004) 'The Path-Dependency of an Idea: Why Scandinavian Welfare States Remain Distinct', *Social Policy and Administration*, 38(2), 204–219

Dahlström, C. et al (2020) 'Conflict-Resolvers or Tools of Electoral Struggle? Swedish Commissions of Inquiry 1990–2016', *Working Paper*, 3, Gothenburg, QOG

Demker, M. (2014), *Sverige åt Svenskarna: Motstånd och Mobilisering mot Invandring och Invandrare i Sverige*, Stockholm, Atlas

Economist, The (2013) 'The Next Supermodel', *The Economist*, [online] 2 February, www.economist.com/leaders/2013/02/02/the-next-supermodel

Edwards, E. (2020) 'Fauci, Paul Clash over Covid-19 Herd Immunity', *NBC News*, [online] 23 September, www.nbcnews.com/health/health-news/fauci-paul-clash-over-covid-19-herd-immunity-senate-hearing-n1240858

Elder, N. et al (1982) *The Consensual Democracies: The Government and Politics of the Scandinavian States*, Oxford, Martin Robertson

Elmbrant, B. (2020) 'Så synliggjorde Klassamhället', *Dagens Arena*, [online] 21 July, www.dagensarena.se/essa/sa-synliggjorde-coronan-klassamhallet/

Emmeneger, P. et al (eds) (2012) *The Age of Dualization: The Changing Face of Inequality in Deindustrializing Societies*, Oxford, Oxford University Press

Engberg, K. (2004) *När Totalförsvaret Föll Samman*, Stockholm, Kungliga Krigsvetenskapsakademin

Erdbrink, T. (2020) 'Sweden Tries Out a New Status: Pariah State', *The New York Times*, [online] 22 June, www.nytimes.com/2020/06/22/world/europe/sweden-coronavirus-pariah-scandinavia.html

Eriksson, G. (2020a) 'Folkhälsonationalism kan förklara den svenska linjen', *Svenska Dagbladet*, [online], www.svd.se/folkhalsonationalism-kan-forklara-svenska-coronalinjen

Eriksson, G. (2020b) 'Sverige har haft för dåligt beredskap', *Svenska Dagbladet*, [online] 9 April, www.svd.se/stefan-lofven-vi-har-inte-lyckats-skydda-vara-aldre

Eriksson, G. (2020c) 'Så har coronaviruset gjort Sverige stort igen', *Svenska Dagbladet*, [online] 25 April, www.svd.se/sa-har-coronaviruset-gjort-sverige-stort-igen

Eriksson, G. et al (2020) 'Så föddes Sveriges coronaplan: Spelet bakom kulisserna', *Svenska Dagbladet*, [online] 5 July, www.svd.se/forbered-er-pa-det-varsta--spelet-bakom-coronastrategin

Erlandsson, Å and Eriksson, H. (2020) 'Överläkaren: Vi vill inte ha fältssjukhuset i Älvsjö', *Svenska Dagbladet*, [online] 26 May, www.svd.se/overlakaren-vi-ville-inte-ha-faltsjukhuset-i-alvsjo

Esping-Andersen, G. (1985) *Politics Against Markets*, Princeton, Princeton University Press

Esping-Andersen, G. (1990) *The Three Worlds of Welfare Capitalism*, Princeton, Princeton University Press

Ezensberger, H-M. (1982) *Svensk höst*, Stockholm, Dagens Nyheter

Falkirk, J. (2020) 'Norska kritiken: "Giesecke borde vara mer ödmjuk"', *Svenska Dagbladet*, [online] 16 May, www.svd.se/norska-kritiken-giesecke-borde-vara-mer-odmjuk

Fenwick Elliott, A. (2020) 'Sweden's Resistance Raises Questions About Our Own Tough Approach', *The Telegraph*, [online] 27 March, www.telegraph.co.uk/news/2020/03/27/swedens-resistance-lockdown-raises-questions-tough-approach/

Ferguson, N. et al (2020) 'Impact of Non-Pharmaceutical Interventions (NPIs) to Reduce COVID-19 Mortality and Healthcare Demand', *Report n° 16*, London, Imperial College Covid-19 Response Team

Folkhälsomyndigheten (2020) 'Vaccinationstäckning per födelseland, inkomst och utbildningsgrad', [report], www.folkhalsomyndigheten.se/folkhalsorapportering-statistik/statistikdatabaser-och-visualisering/vaccinationsstatistik/statistik-for-vaccination-mot-covid-19/uppfoljning-av-vaccination/vaccinationstackning-i-undergrupper/

Folkhälsomyndigheten (2021) 'Undersökning om acceptans för vaccination mot covid-19 – Resultat mars 2021', [report], www.folkhalsomyndigheten.se/smittskydd-beredskap/utbrott/aktuella-utbrott/covid-19/statistik-och-analyser/acceptans-for-vaccination-mot-covid-19/resultat-mars-2021/

Forsberg, O. (2020) 'Tegnell om danskbeslut: "Fullständigt meningslös åtgärd"', *Aftonbladet*, [online] 13 March, www.aftonbladet.se/nyheter/a/9vdeo9/tegnell-om-danskbeslut-fullstandigt-meningslos-atgard

Freeman, R.B. et al (eds) *Reforming the Welfare State: Recovery and Beyond in Sweden*, Chicago, University of Chicago Press

Friedman, T.L. (2020) 'Is Sweden Getting It Right with Its COVID-19 Approach?', *Mercury News*, [online], www.mercurynews.com/2020/04/30/friedman-is-sweden-getting-it-right-with-its-covid-19-approach/

Fukuyama, F. (2011) *The Origins of Political Order*, New York, Farrar, Straus and Giroux

Gaille, M. and Terral, P. (2021) *Pandémie: Un Fait Social Total*, Paris, CNRS Editions

Garcia, J. et al (2021) 'Differences in COVID-19 Mortality: Implications of Imperfect and Diverse Data Collection Systems', *Population-E*, 76(1), 35–72, www.cairn-int.info/load_pdf.php?ID_ARTICLE=E_POPU_2101_0037&download=1

Gaudillière, J-P. et al (2021) *Pandémopolitique: Réinventer la santé en commun*, Paris, La Découverte

Geoghegan, P. (2021) 'Now the Swedish Model Has Failed, It's Time to Ask Who Was Pushing It', *The Guardian*, [online] 3 January, www.theguardian.com/commentisfree/2021/jan/03/swedish-model-failed-covid-19

Giesecke, J. (2020) 'De Flesta kommer att smittas', *Svenska Dagbladet*, [online] 6 May, www.svd.se/giesecke-de-flesta-kommer-att-smittas

Gjerde, L.E.L (2020) 'From Liberalism to Biopolitics: Investigating the Norwegian Government's Two Responses to Covid-19', *European Societies*, 23:sup1, 262–274, http://Doi:10.1080/14616696.2020.1824003

Glover, N. (2015) 'A Total Image Deconstructed: The Corporate Analogy and the Legitimacy of Promoting Sweden Abroad in the 1960s', in L. Clerc et al (eds) *Histories of Public Diplomacy and Nation Branding in the Nordic and Baltic Countries. Representing the Periphery*, Leiden, Brill, 123–144

Goodman, P.S. (2020) 'Sweden Has Become the World's Cautionary Tale', *The New York Times*, [online] 7 July, www.nytimes.com/2020/07/07/business/sweden-economy-coronavirus.html

Götz, N. and Marklund, C. (eds) (2015) *The Paradox of Openness: Transparency and Participation in Nordic Cultures of Consensus*, Leiden, Brill

Granberg, M. et al (2021) 'Debate: Covid-19 and Sweden's Exceptionalism – a Spotlight on the Cracks in the Social Fabric of a Mature Welfare State', *Public Money & Management*, 41(3), 223–224, http://Doi: 10.1080/09540962.2020.1866842

Gras, A. (2020) 'Le modèle de la Suède non confinée à l'heure du déconfinement', *Libération.fr*, [online] 5 June, www.liberation.fr/debats/2020/05/06/le-modele-de-la-suede-non-confinee-a-l-heure-du-deconfinement_1787446/

Greene, A. (2020) *Emergency Powers in a Time of Pandemic*, Bristol, Bristol University Press

Greer, S.L. et al (2020) *Coronavirus Politics: The Comparative Politics and Policy of Covid-19*, Ann Arbor, University of Michigan Press.

Greve, B. (2020) *Welfare, Populism and Welfare Chauvinism*, Bristol, Policy Press

Greve, B. et al (2020) 'Nordic Welfare States: Still Standing or Changed by the Covid Crisis?' *Social Policy & Administration*, 55(2), 295–311, www.ncbi.nlm.nih.gov/pmc/articles/PMC7753633/

Grothe-Hammer, M. and Roth, S. (2020) 'Dying Is Normal, Dying with the Coronavirus Is Not: A Sociological Analysis of the Implicit Norms Behind the Criticism of Swedish "Exceptionalism"', *European Societies*, 23:sup1, 332–347, http://Doi:10.1080/14616696.2020.1826555

Gustavsson, G. and Miller, D. (2019) *Liberal Nationalism and its Critics: Normative and Empirical Questions*, Oxford, Oxford University Press

Harvey, O. (2020) 'Hero Swede: How Ice Cool Scientist Saved Sweden from Coronavirus Without Lockdown', *The Sun*, [online] 18 September, www.thesun.co.uk/news/12710684/anders-tegnell-scientist-sweden-coronavirus-without-lockdown-national-hero/

Heldahl, E.H. 'Kritik av äldreomsorgen begravdes i ett bergsrum', *Dagens Nyheter*, [online] 18 December, www.dn.se/debatt/kritik-av-aldreomsorgen-begravdes-i-ett-bergrum/

Helsingen, L.M. et al (2020) 'The COVID-19 Pandemic in Norway and Sweden – Threats, Trust, and Impact on Daily Life: A Comparative Survey', *BMC Public Health*, 20(1597), https://doi.org/10.1186/s12889-020-09615-3

Henley, J. (2020a) 'Swedish PM Warned Over "Russian Roulette-Style" Covid-19 Strategy', *The Guardian*, [online] 23 March, www.theguardian.com/world/2020/mar/23/swedish-pm-warned-russian-roulette-covid-19-strategy-herd-immunity

Henley, J. (2020b) 'Just 7.3% of Stockholm Had Covid-19 Antibodies by End of April, Study Shows', *The Guardian*, [online] 21 May, www.theguardian.com/world/2020/may/21/just-7-per-cent-of-stockholm-had-covid-19-antibodies-by-end-of-april-study-sweden-coronavirus

Hennette-Vauchez, S. (2022) *La démocratie en état d'urgence: Quand l'exception devient permanente*, Paris, Seuil.

Hilson, M. (2008) *The Nordic Model: Scandinavia Since 1945*, London, Reaktion Books

Hirdman, Y. (1989) *Att Lägga Livet till Rätta*, Stockholm, Carlsson

Hivert, A-F. (2020a) 'Coronavirus: en Suède, des mesures qui semblent dérisoires comparées à celles d'autres pays', *Le Monde*, [online] 18 March, www.lemonde.fr/planete/article/2020/03/18/la-suede-en-decalage-sur-la-gestion-du-coronavirus_6033528_3244.html

Hivert, A-F. (2020b) 'Les immigrés installés en Suède sont les premiers frappés par le coronavirus', *Le Monde*, [online] 25 March, www.lemonde.fr/international/article/2020/03/25/les-immigres-installes-en-suede-premiers-frappes-par-le-coronavirus_6034429_3210.html

Holt, E. (2018) 'Health in Sweden: A Political Issue', *The Lancet*, 392(10154), 1184–1185, https://doi.org/10.1016/S0140-6736(18)32459-0

Horton, R. (2020) 'Covid-19 Is Not a Pandemic', *The Lancet*, 396(10255), 874, https://doi.org/10.1016/S0140-6736(20)32000-6

Huntford, R. (1971) *The New Totalitarians*, London, Allen Lane

Huupponen, M. (2020) *Pandemi På Äldreboende*, [trade union report], Kommunal

Ingebritsen, C. (2006) *Scandinavia in World Politics*, Lanham, Rowman & Littlefield

Ingimundarson, V. et al (2016) *Iceland's Financial Crisis: The Politics of Blame, Protest, and Reconstruction*, London, Routledge

Inspektionen för Vård och Omsorg (IVO) (2020) *Vad har IVO sett 2020* [report], Stockholm

Irwin, R.E. (2019) 'Sweden's Engagement in Global Health: A Historical Review', *Global Health*, 15(79) https://doi.org/10.1186/s12992-019-0499-1

Irwin, R.E. (2020) 'Misinformation and De-Contextualization: International Media Reporting on Sweden and COVID-19', *Global Health*, 16(1), www.ncbi.nlm.nih.gov/pmc/articles/PMC7356107/

Jacquin, J-B. (2020) 'Coronavirus: L'état d'urgence sanitaire ouvre des brèches dans l'Etat de droit', *Lemonde.fr*, [online] 28 March, www.lemonde.fr/societe/article/2020/03/28/coronavirus-l-etat-d-urgence-sanitaire-ouvre-des-breches-dans-l-etat-de-droit_6034751_3224.html

Jakobsen, S.E. and Amundsen, B. (2021) 'Hvorfor valgte Sverige en mere dødelig corona-strategi end Danmark og Norge?', *Videnskab.dk*, [online] 11 March, https://videnskab.dk/kultur-samfund/hvorfor-valgte-sverige-en-mere-doedelig-corona-strategi-end-danmark-og-norge

Jonasson, P. and Larue, T. (2020) 'La pandémie de Covid-19 et le Parlement suédois: comment utiliser un cadre constitutionnel flexible', [report], Fondation Robert Schuman

Jonsson-Cornell, A. and Salminen, J. (2018) 'Emergency Laws in Comparative Constitutional Law – The Case of Sweden and Finland', German Law Journal, 19(2), 219–250, http://doi:10.1017/S2071832200022677

Jonung, L. (2020) 'Sweden's Constitution Decides Its Exceptional Covid-19 Policy', *Voxeu.org*, [online] 18 June, https://voxeu.org/article/sweden-s-constitution-decides-its-exceptional-covid-19-policy

JustitieOmbudsmän (JO) (2020) *Yttrande över promemorian Covid-19-lag*, [report] 18 December, https://www.jo.se/Global/Remissyttranden/Remissyttrande%20R_144-2020.pdf

Juul, F. et al (2020) 'Mortality in Norway and Sweden Before and After the Covid-19 Outbreak: A Cohort Study', *medRxiv*, 11 November, https://doi.org/10.1101/2020.11.11.20229708

Kamali, M. and Jönsson, J.H. (eds) (2018) *Neoliberalism and Social Work in the Nordic Welfare States*, London, Routledge

Kananen, J. (2016) *The Nordic Welfare State in Three Eras: From Emancipation to Discipline*, London, Routledge

Katz, D.L. (2020) 'Is Our Fight Against Coronavirus Worse Than the Disease?', *The New York Times*, [online] 20 March, www.nytimes.com/2020/03/20/opinion/coronavirus-pandemic-social-distancing.html

Kennedy, R. (2020) 'Coronavirus: Nigel Farage Cites Sweden as He Relaunches Brexit Party to Oppose COVID-19 Lockdowns', *Euronews*, [online] 2 November, www.euronews.com/2020/11/02/coronavirus-nigel-farage-cites-sweden-as-he-relaunches-brexit-party-to-oppose-covid-19-loc

Kettunen, P. and Petersen, K. (2022) 'Images of the Nordic Welfare Model: Historical Layers and Ambiguities', in H. Byrkjeflot et al (eds) *The Making and Circulation of Nordic Models, Ideas and Images*, London, Routledge, 13–34

Keussen, E. et al (2020) 'Regeringen blunder för fakta om äldreomsorgen', *Debatt*, [online] 12 July, www.expressen.se/debatt/sju-chefer-for-aldreboenden-regeringen-har-blundat-for-fakta/

King, D. and Le Galès, P. (2017) *Reconfiguring European States in Crisis*, Oxford, Oxford University Press.

Klitgaard, M.B. (2007) 'Why Are They Doing it? Social Democracy and Market-Oriented Welfare State Reforms', *West European Politics*, 30(1), 172–194, https://Doi:10.1080/01402380601019753

Knight, D.R. (2021) 'New Zealand: Rendering Account During the COVID-19 Pandemic', *Verfasssungsblog*, [online], https://verfassungsblog.de/new-zealand-rendering-account-during-the-covid-19-pandemic/

Kullberg, F. (2020) 'Hon är doldisen som leder regeringens krisgrupp', *Chef*, [online] 11 May, https://chef.se/hon-ar-doldisen-som-leder-regeringens-krisgrupp/

Kumlin, S. and Haugsgjerd, A. (2017) 'The Welfare State and Political Trust: Bringing Performance Back In', in S. Zmerli and T.W.G. van der Meer (eds) *Handbook on Political Trust*, Cheltenham, Edward Elgar Publishing, 285–301

Landström, R. (2020) *Coronateserna*, Stockholm, Verbal Förlag

Laurén, A-L. (2020) 'Intresset för Sverige har ökat under coronapandemin', *Dagens Nyheter*, [online] 2 June, www.dn.se/nyheter/varlden/intresset-for-sverige-har-okat-under-coronapandemin

Liljestrand, J. (2020) 'Anders Tegnell ä den svenska nasjonalsjälen förkroppsligad', *Expressen*, [online] 15 April, www.expressen.se/kronikorer/jens-liljestrand/anders-tegnell-ar-den-svenska-nationalsjalen-forkroppsligad/

Liman, L. and Rolander, N. (2020) 'Swedish COVID Expert Says the World Still Doesn't Understand', *The National Post*, [online] 30 June, https://nationalpost.com/news/canada/swedish-covid-expert-says-the-world-still-doesnt-understand

Lindberg, S. (2020a) 'Dokument avslöjar: Så försöker regeringen rädda Sverigebilden', *Aftonbladet*, [online] 2 June, www.aftonbladet.se/nyheter/a/kJ75LQ/dokument-avslojar-sa-forsoker-regeringen-radda-sverigebilden

Lindberg, A. (2020b) 'Sverige borde införa ministerstyre i kriser', *Aftonbladet*, [online] 21 June, www.aftonbladet.se/ledare/a/0n5Mwg/sverige-borde-infora-ministerstyre-i-kriser

Lindbom, A. (2001) 'Dismantling the Social Democratic Welfare Model? Has the Swedish Welfare State Lost Its Defining Characteristics?', *Scandinavian Political Studies*, 24(3), 171–193, https://doi.org/10.1111/1467-9477.00052

Lindgren, L. et al (2020) 'Tegnells teori får stöd – men andra är tveksamma', *Aftonbladet*, [online] 18 September, www.aftonbladet.se/nyheter/a/mB63GO/tegnells-teori-far-stod--men-andra-ar-tveksamma

Lindström, M. (2020) 'The New Totalitarians: The Swedish COVID-19 Strategy and the Implications of Consensus Culture and Media Policy for Public Health', *Population Health*, 14, https://doi.org/10.1016/j.ssmph.2021.100788

Löfgren, E. (2020) '"The Biggest Challenge of Our Time': How Sweden Doubled Intensive Care Capacity Amid Covid-19 Pandemic', *The Local*, [online] 23 June, www.thelocal.com/20200623/how-sweden-doubled-intensive-care-capacity-to-treat-coronavirus-patients/

Lund, L. (2020a) 'Så ser omvärlden på den svenska "experimentet"', *Dagens Nyheter*, [online] 25 March, www.dn.se/nyheter/varlden/sa-ser-omvarlden-pa-det-svenska-experimentet/

Lund, L. (2020b) 'Vem är tysken som ställer Tegnell mot väggen?', *Dagens Nyheter*, [online] 1 April, www.dn.se/nyheter/sverige/vem-ar-tysken-som-staller-tegnell-mot-vaggen/

Lund, L. (2020c) 'Schweden ses inte längre som en "bullerbyidyll" i Tyskland', *Dagens Nyheter*, [online] 2 June, www.dn.se/nyheter/varlden/schweden-ses-inte-langre-som-en-bullerbyidyll-i-tyskland

Lundqvist, Å. and Petersen, K. (2010) *In Experts We Trust: Knowledge and Bureaucracy in Nordic Welfare States*, Odense, University Press of Southern Denmark.

Mai, H.J. (2020) 'Swedish Ambassador Says Stockholm Expected to Reach "Herd Immunity" in May', *NPR*, [online] 26 April, www.npr.org/2020/04/26/845211085/stockholm-expected-to-reach-herd-immunity-in-may-swedish-ambassador-says

Mandavili, A. (2021) 'Reaching "Herd Immunity" Is Unlikely in the U.S., Experts Now Believe', *The New York Times*, [online] 3 May, www.nytimes.com/2021/05/03/health/covid-herd-immunity-vaccine.html

Mann, T. (2020) 'Sweden's Coronavirus Plan Failed to Stop the Virus, and a Vaccine May Not Be Enough to "Rescue" Them, Experts Warn', *ABC News*, [online] 27 November, www.abc.net.au/news/2020-11-28/sweden-paid-too-high-a-price-with-its-rogue-coronavirus-policy/12922932

Marklund, C. (2009) 'Hot Love and Cold People Sexual Liberalism as Political Escapism in Radical Sweden', *NORDEUROPAforum – Zeitschrift für Kulturstudien*, 19(1), 83–101, https://Doi:10.18452/7999

Marklund, C. (2016) 'The Nordic Model on the Global Market of Ideas: The Welfare State as Scandinavia's Best Brand', *Geopolitics*, 22(3), 1–17, https://Doi:10.1080/14650045.2016.1251906

Milne, R. (2020) 'Anders Tegnell and the Swedish Covid Experiment', *Financial Times*, [online] 11 September, www.ft.com/content/5cc92d45-fbdb-43b7-9c66-26501693a371

Moe, I. (2021b) 'De forsker på Norden under koronaen: Derfor var det ikke snakk om dugnad i Sverige', *Aftenposten*, [online] 7 July, www.aftenposten.no/verden/i/GazK3l/de-forsker-paa-norden-under-koronaen-derfor-var-det-ikke-snakk-om-dugn

Moreira, A. and Hick, R. (2021) 'COVID-19, the Great Recession and Social Policy: Is This Time Different?', *Social Policy & Administration*, 55(2), 261–279, https://doi.org/10.1111/spol.12679

Morel, N. et al (eds) (2011) *Toward a Social Investment Welfare State? Ideas, Policies and Challenges*, Bristol, Policy Press

Musial, K. (2002) *Roots of the Scandinavian Model: Images of Progress in the Era of Modernisation*, Baden-Baden, Nomos Verlag

Nelson, F. (2020) 'Sweden, Covid and Lockdown – A Look at the Data', *The Spectator*, [online] 16 May, www.spectator.co.uk/article/sweden-covid-and-lockdown-a-look-at-the-data

Nelson, K. (2017) 'Lower Unemployment Benefits and Old-Age Pensions Is a Major Setback in Social Policy', *Sociologisk Forskning*, 54 (4), 287–291, www.jstor.org/stable/26632197

Nguyen, T. (2020) 'Conservative Americans See Coronavirus Hope in Progressive Sweden', *Politico*, [online] 30 April, www.politico.com/news/2020/04/30/conservative-coronavirus-sweden-225184

Nilsson, A-S. (1991) *Den Moraliska Stormakten: En studie av socialdemokratins internationella aktivism*, Stockholm, Timbro

Nott, K. (1961) *A Clean, Well-Lighted Place: A Private View of Sweden*, London, Heinemann

Orange, R. (2020a) 'Anger in Sweden as Elderly Pay Price for Coronavirus Strategy', *The Guardian*, [online] 19 April, www.theguardian.com/world/2020/apr/19/anger-in-sweden-as-elderly-pay-price-for-coronavirus-strategy

Orange, R. (2020b) 'Inside the City that May Prove the Country's Strategy Was Right All Along', *The Telegraph*, [online] 14 June, www.telegraph.co.uk/news/2020/06/14/inside-swedish-city-may-prove-countrys-strategy-right-along/

Osborne, S. (2020) 'Sweden's Top Epidemiologist Explains Country's "Trust Based" Approach to Tackling Coronavirus', *The Independent*, [online] 24 April, www.independent.co.uk/news/world/europe/sweden-coronavirus-lockdown-cases-deaths-schools-bars-restaurants-open-a9482236.html

Palm, E.A. (2020) 'Swedish Exceptionalism Has Been Ended by Coronavirus', *The Guardian*, [online] 26 June, www.theguardian.com/commentisfree/2020/jun/26/swedish-exceptionalism-coronavirus-covid19-death-toll

Pancevski, B. (2020) 'Long a Holdout from Covid-19 Restrictions, Sweden Ends Its Pandemic Experiment', *The Wall Street Journal*, [online] 6 December, www.wsj.com/articles/long-a-holdout-from-covid-19-restrictions-sweden-ends-its-pandemic-experiment-11607261658

Persson, L. and Sjöholm, F. (2021) 'Coronastrategin har varit bra för svensk ekonomi', *Dagens Nyheter*, [online] 8 March, www.dn.se/debatt/coronastrategin-har-varit-bra-for-svensk-ekonomi/

Pieper, D. (2020) 'Die schwedische Enttäuschung', *Spiegel Ausland*, [online] 20 December, www.spiegel.de/ausland/corona-horror-in-schweden-erfahrungen-in-einem-einstigen-traumland-a-1f71fbef-6009-4562-af5d-653a371802d6

Pierre, J. (2020) 'Nudges Against Pandemics: Sweden's COVID-19 Containment Strategy in Perspective', *Policy and Society*, 29(3), 478–493, https://doi.org/10.1080/14494035.2020.1783787

Pontusson, J. (2005) *Inequality and Prosperity: Social Europe vs Liberal America*, Ithaca, Cornell University Press.

Ramesh, R. (2012) 'Private Healthcare: The Lessons from Sweden', *The Guardian*, [online] 18 December, www.theguardian.com/society/2012/dec/18/private-healthcare-lessons-from-sweden

Rapacioli, P. (2018a) 'Det goda Sverige vs det dåliga Sverige: Sverigebilden som vapen i ideologiska strider' in J. Andersson Schwarz et al *Sverigebilden. On journalistik och verklighet*, Stockholm, Institut för mediestudier, 81–99

Rapacioli, P. (2018b) *Good Sweden, Bad Sweden: The Use and Abuse of Swedish Values in a Post-Truth World*, Stockholm, Volante

Rolander, N. (2020) 'Swedish Vaccine Skepticism Is Latest Obstacle to Herd Immunity', *Bloomberg*, [online] 4 December, www.bloomberg.com/news/articles/2020-12-04/sweden-unveils-vaccine-strategy-after-26-reject-immunization

Röstlund, L. and Gustafsson, A. (2020) 'Läkare: Vi tvingas till hårda prioriteringar', *Dagens Nyheter*, [online] 24 April, www.dn.se/sthlm/lakare-vi-tvingas-till-harda-prioriteringar/

Rothstein, B. (1998) *Just Institutions Matter: The Moral and Political Logic of the Universal Welfare State*, Harvard, Cambridge University Press

Rothstein, B. (2020) 'Regeringens styrning har inte fungerat i coronakrisen', *Dagens Nyheter*, [online] 30 November, www.dn.se/debatt/regeringens-styrning-har-inte-fungerat-i-coronakrisen/

Ryner, M.J. (2002) *Capitalist Restructuring, Globalization and the Third Way: Lessons from the Swedish Model*, London, Routledge

Sadikovic, A. and Ridderstedt, M. (2020) 'Anhöriga: Vi involverades inte i livsavgörande beslut', *Sveriges Radio*, [online] 29 September, https://sverigesradio.se/artikel/7561304

Sample, I. (2020) 'Covid: Ministers Ignored Sage Advice to Impose Lockdown or Face Catastrophe', *The Guardian*, [online] 13 October, www.theguardian.com/world/2020/oct/12/ministers-rejected-four-out-five-proposals-from-sage-to-avert-covid-second-wave

Savage, M. (2020) 'Coronavirus: What's Going Wrong in Sweden's Care Homes?', *BBC News*, [online] 19 May, www.bbc.com/news/world-europe-52704836

Sayers, F. (2020) 'Swedish Expert: Why Lockdowns Are the Wrong Policy', *Unherd*, [online] 17 April, https://unherd.com/thepost/coming-up-epidemiologist-prof-johan-giesecke-shares-lessons-from-sweden

Sellström, T. (1999) *Sweden and National Liberation in Southern Africa*, Uppsala, Nordiska Afrikainstitutet

Selnes, A. (2021) 'Svensk a-kassa bland de lägsta i EU', *Europaportalen*, [online] 31 May, www.europaportalen.se/2021/05/svenskt-kassa-bland-de-lagsta-i-eu

Servan-Schreiber, J-J. (1968) *Le Défi Américain*, Paris, Denoël

Shilton, J. (2020) 'Architect of Sweden's Coronavirus Policy Advocated Keeping Schools Open to Reach "Herd Immunity" More Quickly', *WSWS.org*, [online] 21 August, www.wsws.org/en/articles/2020/08/21/tegn-a21.html

Simons, G. (2020) 'Swedish Government and Country Image During the International Media Coverage of the Coronavirus Pandemic Strategy: from Bold to Pariah', *Journalism and Media*, 1, 41–58, doi:10.3390/journalmedia1010004

Stichler, C. (2020) 'Coronavirus: Die Welt steht still. Nur Schweden nicht', *Die Zeit*, [online] 24 March, www.zeit.de/zustimmung?url=https%3A%2F%2Fwww.zeit.de%2Fpolitik%2Fausland%2F2020-03%2Fcoronavirus-schweden-stockholm-oeffentliches-leben

Stiegler, B. (2020) *De la Démocratie en Pandémie*, Paris, Gallimard

Stolt, R. and Winblad, U. (2009) 'Mechanisms Behind Privatization: A Case Study of Private Growth in Swedish Elderly Care', *Social Science & Medicine*, 68(5), 903–911

Stråth, B. (2006) 'La construction d'un modèle nordique: pressions externes et compromis internes', *Revue internationale de politique comparée*, 13(3), 391–411

Stråth, B. (2012) 'Nordic Modernity: Origins, Trajectories, Perspectives', in J. Páll Árnason and B. Wittrock (eds) *Nordic Paths to Modernity*, New York, Berghahn Books, 25–49

Strittmatter, K. (2020) 'Das nächste Ischgl', *Süddeutsche Zeitung*, [online] 22 March, www.sueddeutsche.de/panorama/coronavirus-are-schweden-skigebiet-1.4853632

Suhonen, D. (2020) Vi mötte tyvärr inte corona tillsammans, *Aftonbladet*, [online] 29 May, www.aftonbladet.se/ledare/a/Opv9aO/vi-motte-tyvarr-inte-corona-tillsammans

Sulyok, M. and Walker, M.D. (2021) 'Mobility and COVID-19 Mortality Across Scandinavia: A Modeling Study', *Travel Med Infect Dis*, 41, doi:10.1016/j.tmaid.2021.102039

Svallfors, S. (2011) 'A Bedrock of Support? Trends in Welfare State Attitudes in Sweden, 1981–2010', *Social Policy & Administration*, 45(7), 806–825, https://doi.org/10.1111/j.1467-9515.2011.00796.x

Svenska Institutet (2020) *Samtalet om Sverige*, Stockholm, https://si.se/app/uploads/2021/02/samtalet-om-sverige-2020-04-08.pdf

Tarquini, A. (2020) 'Coronavirus, la Svezia va controcorrente: mezzi di trasporto pieni e uffici aperti', *La Repubblica*, [online] 26 March, www.repubblica.it/esteri/2020/03/26/news/coronavirus_la_svezia_va_controcorrente_mezzi_di_trasporto_pieni_e_uffici_aperti-252380584/

Tassinari, F. (2020) 'A Tale of Two Pandemics', *Noema*, [online] 12 November, www.noemamag.com/a-tale-of-two-pandemics/

Thelen, K. (2014)a *Varieties of Liberalization and the New Politics of Social Solidarity*, Cambridge, Cambridge University Press.

Trägårdh, L. (1997) 'Statist Institutionalism: on the Culturality of the Nordic Welfare State', in Ø. Sørensen and B. Stråth (eds) *The Cultural Construction of Norden*, Oslo, SUP

Trägårdh, L. (2007) 'Democratic Governance and the Creation of Social Capital in Sweden: The Discreet Charm of Governmental Commissions', in L. Trägårdh (ed) *State and Civil Society in Northern Europe. The Swedish Model Reconsidered*, New York, Berghahn Books, 254–271

Trägårdh, L. (2018) 'Granskninsamhället i högtillitslandet Sverige', in L. Bringselius (ed) *Styra och Leda med Tillit: Forskning och Praktik*, Stockholm, SOU 38, 406–425

Trägårdh, L. (2020) 'La Suède lutte contre la pandémie due au coronavirus à travers la "liberté sous responsabilité"', *Le Monde*, [online] 10 April, www.lemonde.fr/international/article/2020/04/10/lars-tragardh-la-suede-lutte-contre-la-pandemie-a-travers-la-liberte-sous-responsabilite_6036233_3210.html

Trägårdh, L. and Özkirimli, U. (2020) 'Why Might Sweden's Covid-19 Policy Work? Trust Between Citizens and State', *The Guardian*, [online] 21 April, www.theguardian.com/world/commentisfree/2020/apr/21/sweden-covid-19-policy-trust-citizens-state

Truedsson, L. (2018) 'Kampen om Sverigebilden', in J. Andersson Schwarz et al (eds) *Sverigebilden: On journalistik och verklighet*, Stockholm, Institut för mediestudier, 7–15

Tubilewicz, K. (2020) 'Sverige har förblivit envist fritt i pandemin', *Kvartal*, [online] 20 December, https://kvartal.se/artiklar/sverige-har-forblivit-envist-fritt-i-pandemin

Unherd (2020) 'Norwegian Health Chief: We Advised Against Closing Schools', *Unherd*, [online] 10 June, https://unherddev.wpengine.com/thepost/norwegian-health-chief-we-advised-against-closing-schools/

Von Hall, U. (2021) ' "Nörden" som blev hela Sveriges vaccingeneral', *Svenska Dagbladet*, [online] 18 July, www.svd.se/norden-som-blev-hela-sveriges-vaccingeneral

Widfeldt, A. (2018) 'The Radical Right in the Nordic Countries', in J. Rydgren (ed) *The Oxford Handbook of the Radical Right*, Oxford, Oxford University Press, 545–565

Wierup, M. and Wågsholm, I. (2020) 'Folkhälsomyndighetens två uppdrag är oförenliga', *Dagens Nyheter*, [online] 28 November, www.dn.se/debatt/folkhalsomyndighetens-tva-uppdrag-ar-oforenliga/

Wiman, B. (2020) 'Så döljer folkhemmets fasad coronastrategins baksida', *Dagens Nyheter*, [online] 16 May, www.dn.se/kultur-noje/bjorn-wiman-sa-doljer-folkhemmets-fasad-coronastrategins-baksida/

Wolodarski, P. (2020a) 'Ursäkta, måste vi vara plågsamt långsamma?', *Dagens Nyheter*, [online] 8 March, www.dn.se/ledare/peter-wolodarski-ursakta-maste-vi-vara-plagsamt-langsamma/

Wolodarski, P. (2020b) 'Stäng ner Sverige för att skydda Sverige', *Dagens Nyheter*, [online] 13 March, www.dn.se/ledare/peter-wolodarski-stang-ned-sverige-for-att-skydda-sverige/

Wondmeneh, Y. (2013) *Mångfald i Äldreomsorgen*, Stockholm, Kommunal

Wooler, S. (2020) 'Stockholm Syndrome', *The Sun*, [online] 3 June, www.thesun.co.uk/news/11769567/neil-ferguson-praises-sweden-lockdown/

Woolhouse, M. (2020) 'Lockdown Failed: We Must Follow the Swedish Model and Learn to Live with Covid', *The Telegraph*, [online] 19 September, www.telegraph.co.uk/news/2020/09/19/uk-needs-follow-swedish-model-learn-live-covid/

Zangana, B. (2020) 'Tegnell om uttalandet: "Det var olyckligt"', *Aftonbladet*, [online] 4 December, www.aftonbladet.se/nyheter/a/gW3E1A/tegnell-om-uttalandet-det-var-olyckligt

Zølck, J. (2020) 'Sverige forsvarer sin corona-strategi: Vi undrer os også over Danmark', *TV2*, [online] 30 March, https://nyheder.tv2.dk/udland/2020-03-30-sverige-forsvarer-sin-corona-strategi-vi-undrer-os-ogsaa-over-danmark

Index

Page numbers in *italic* type refer to figures.
Reference to endnotes show both the
page number and the note number (231n3).

Printed and bound by CPI Group (UK) Ltd, Croydon, CR0 4YY

07/07/2026

14916219-0003